Glencoe

Computers in the
Medical Office

Using MediSoft for Windows

With Student Data Disk

Susan M. Sanderson

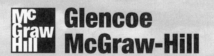

**Glencoe
McGraw-Hill**

New York, New York
Columbus, Ohio
Woodland Hills, California
Peoria, Illinois

Library of Congress Cataloging-in-Publication Data

Sanderson, Susan M.
   Computers in the medical office : using MediSoft for Windows/Susan
M. Sanderson.
   p.   cm.

   ISBN 0-02-801990-3 (pb)
   1. Medical offices—Automation.- 2. MediSoft.
R864.C656   1999
651'.961' 0285—dc21   97-43098
                                                         CIP

Glencoe/McGraw-Hill

A Division of The **McGraw·Hill** Companies

Send all inquiries to:
Glencoe/McGraw-Hill
8787 Orion Place
Columbus, OH 43240

ISBN 0-02-801990-3

  5 6 7 8 9   066   05 04 03 02 01 00 99

Codeveloped by
Glencoe/McGraw-Hill
and Chestnut Hill Enterprises, Inc.
Woodbury, CT

The Student Data Disk, illustrations, instructions, and exercises in *Computers in the Medical Office:
Using MediSoft for Windows* are compatible with the MediSoft Patient Accounting for Windows
software available at the time of publication. Adaptations may be necessary for use with
subsequent versions of the software. Text changes will be made in reprints when possible.

Contents

Preface

Demand for health care services is increasing, due to technological advances and to an aging population. Administrative duties in medical offices are also becoming more involved with technology. Computers are playing an ever-increasing role in helping to handle some of the most important functions. Students who aim to find an administrative job in the health care industry will find that computer knowledge is often a prerequisite for employment.

This text/workbook, *Glencoe Computers in the Medical Office: Using MediSoft for Windows*, prepares students for administrative tasks in health care practices. The text/workbook introduces and simulates situations using MediSoft for Windows, a widely used medical administrative software. While progressing through MediSoft's menus and windows, students learn to input patient information, schedule appointments, and handle billing. In addition, they produce various lists and reports, and learn to handle insurance claims both on paper forms and electronically. These invaluable skills are important in effective financial management of health care practices.

Although this text/workbook features MediSoft for Windows, its concepts are general enough to cover most administrative software intended for health care providers. Students who complete *Glencoe Computers in the Medical Office: Using MediSoft for Windows* should be able to use other medical administrative software with a minimum of training.

TEXT/WORKBOOK OVERVIEW

Glencoe Computers in the Medical Office: Using MediSoft for Windows is divided into four parts. The first, "Introduction to Computers in the Medical Office," covers the general flow of information in a medical office and the role that computers play. It also provides an overview of Microsoft Windows 95 for those students who are not yet computer literate. Instructors may wish to use the first part as a review or, if students have had other courses in computers, they may wish to start directly with Part 2. A test has been provided in the *Instructor's Manual* to determine the level of students' familiarity with computers.

Part 2, "MediSoft for Windows Training," teaches students how to start, input data, and use MediSoft to bill patients, file claims, record data, print reports, and schedule appointments. The sequence takes the student through MediSoft for Windows in a clear, concise manner. Each chapter includes a number of exercises that are to be done at the computer. These exercises give the student realistic experience using an administrative medical software program.

Part 3, "Simulations," completes the learning process by requiring the student to perform a series of tasks using MediSoft for Windows. Each task is an application of the knowledge required in the medical office.

At the end of the text/workbook, Part 4, a section of Source Documents, gives the student the data needed to complete the exercises. These forms, including patient information forms and superbills, are similar to those used in medical offices.

COMPUTER SUPPLIES AND EQUIPMENT

The Student Data Disk that comes with the text/workbook provides a base of case study information. Other equipment and supplies needed are as follows:

IBM or IBM-compatible computer
Microsoft Windows 3.1 (or higher) or Windows 95
MediSoft Patient Accounting for Windows 5.2
A blank, formatted, high density 3½" floppy diskette
Printer

MediSoft for Windows is free to schools adopting *Glencoe Computers in the Medical Office: Using MediSoft for Windows*. Information on ordering and installing the software is located in the *Instructor's Manual* that accompanies the text/workbook.

CHAPTER STRUCTURE

At the beginning of each chapter, students are provided with a preview of what will be studied:

What You Need to Know Describes the basic knowledge required in order to complete the chapter.

Objectives Describes the primary areas of knowledge that can be acquired by studying the chapter and performing the exercises.

Key Terms Presents an alphabetic list of important vocabulary terms found in the chapter. Key terms are printed in bold-faced type and defined when introduced in the text. Key term definitions also appear in the left margin of the page where they are first used.

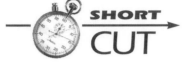

Throughout the instructional chapters, the narrative is supported by numerous figures and tables for reference. These instructional portions of the chapter include *Short Cut* and *Tip* features to enhance the learning experience (see icons in left margin). Computer exercises follow the portions of instructional material to reinforce what was just read.

Various types of testing are supplied in the *Chapter Review* at the end of each chapter in Parts 1 and 2. *Using Terminology* and *Checking Your Understanding* test the student's knowledge of the chapter's key terms and content. *Applying Knowledge* and *At the Computer* encourage the student to use critical thinking skills and apply practical knowledge using the computer.

SUPPLEMENTARY MATERIAL

An *Instructor's Manual* provides the instructor with answers to chapter exercises, answers to Chapter Review questions/exercises, teaching suggestions, a test to help determine the level of students' familiarity with computers, correlation charts for SCANS competencies and foundations as well as the 1997 AAMA Role Delineation Study Areas of Competence, and information on ordering and installing MediSoft for Windows software.

ACKNOWLEDGMENTS

For insightful reviews, criticisms, helpful suggestions, and information, we would like to acknowledge the following:

Deanna Beach
Professional Careers Institute
Indianapolis, Indiana

Karonne Becklin
Anoka-Hennepin Technical College
Anoka, Minnesota

Renae V. Brown
Essex County College
Newark, New Jersey

Anne Conway
National Career Education
Citrus Heights, California

Charlotte Crockett
Morse School of Business
Hartford, Connecticut

Connie L. Greening
Western Career College
Sacramento, California

Marcha Groton
Delaware Technical and Community College, Owens Campus
Georgetown, Delaware

Patti Happel
New England Institute of Technology
West Palm Beach, Florida

Amos C. Jenkins
Southwestern School of Business and Technical Careers
San Antonio, Texas

Deborah Jones
Bryman School
Phoenix, Arizona

Judith Kenyon
San Diego Mesa College
San Diego, California

Gladys Meyer
Plaza Business College
Jackson Heights, New York

Margaret Mott
Wallace Community College Selma
Selma, Alabama

Haig Movsesian
Bryman College
Seatac, Washington

Debra Peelor
Bidwell Training Center, Inc.
Pittsburgh, Pennsylvania

Linda Stanford
McLennan Community College
Waco, Texas

Barbara Tietsort
University of Cincinnati, Raymond Walters College
Cincinnati, Ohio

Dr. Youssef Zakhary
The Cittone Institute
Edison, New Jersey

Introduction to Computers in the Medical Office

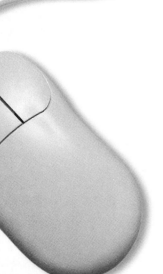

The Flow of Information in the Medical Office

OBJECTIVES

In this chapter, you will learn:

- ◆ The tasks that are performed on a regular basis in the medical office, including scheduling appointments, gathering and recording patient information, recording diagnoses and procedures, billing patients, filing insurance claims, and reviewing and recording payments.
- ◆ The different types of medical insurance.
- ◆ The steps involved in processing claims and collecting payments.

KEY TERMS

coinsurance
copayment
diagnosis
diagnosis code
explanation of benefits (EOB)
Health Insurance Claim
    Form (HCFA-1500)
health maintenance
    organization (HMO)
indemnity plan
insurance carrier

managed care
patient information form
patient statement
policyholder
premiums
procedure code
procedures
providers
schedule of benefits
superbill
third-party payer

THE TASK CYCLE

policyholder *an individual who has contracted with an insurance company for coverage.*

insurance carrier *a company that provides insurance coverage to individuals and/or groups.*

premiums *payments made to an insurance carrier by a policyholder for coverage.*

providers *physicians, hospitals, and other medical staff who provide medical services.*

Most patients are covered by some type of medical insurance. Medical insurance is an agreement between a person, known as the **policyholder**, and an **insurance carrier**. Payments made to the carrier by the policyholder for insurance coverage are called **premiums**. In exchange for these payments, the carrier agrees to pay benefits for medical services. Medical services include care supplied by **providers**—hospitals, physicians, and other medical staff.

From a business standpoint, the key to the financial health of a medical practice is billing and collecting fees for services. Without a steady flow of money coming in, payroll cannot be met, supplies cannot be ordered, the utilities cannot be paid, and so on. To maintain a regular flow of income, certain tasks must be completed in a regular cycle and in a timely manner. These tasks include:

♦ Scheduling appointments

♦ Gathering and recording patient information

♦ Recording diagnoses and procedures

♦ Billing patients and filing insurance claims

♦ Reviewing and recording payments

SCHEDULING APPOINTMENTS

The cycle begins when a patient requests an appointment. New appointment requests are usually made by telephone; follow-up appointments are typically scheduled when the patient is at the front desk, having just seen the physician. When new patients phone for an appointment, they should be informed of the practice's policy regarding payment.

More and more medical offices are using computerized scheduling programs to keep track of patient appointments. If the individual requesting an appointment is an established patient of the practice, the medical office assistant searches for an available time slot that is suitable for the patient and books the appointment. If the individual is a new patient, basic information is recorded (such as the patient's name and phone number) when the appointment is booked. When the new patient arrives at the office for the appointment, additional information is collected. However, in some practices, this additional information is taken over the telephone at the time the appointment is made.

GATHERING AND RECORDING PATIENT INFORMATION

patient information form *a document that contains personal, employment, and medical insurance information about a patient.*

The first time a patient visits the practice, a **patient information form** is completed (see Figure 1-1). The patient information form contains the personal, employment, and medical insurance information needed to file an insurance claim. This form is filed in the patient's medical record and is updated when the patient reports a change, such as a new address. In addition, many offices ask patients to update these forms periodically, to ensure that the information is current and accurate.

Some patient information forms also include miscellaneous information such as:

- ◆ Student status
- ◆ Patient allergies
- ◆ Referring physician
- ◆ Reason for visit
- ◆ Accident information, if appropriate

As shown in Figure 1-1, the patient information form also has places for the patient's signature or for a parent's or guardian's signature if the patient is a minor. One signature authorizes the insurance carrier or governmental program to send payments directly to the provider rather than to the patient. Patients are also asked to sign a release of information statement. This signature gives the medical office permission to release diagnosis and treatment information to the insurance company for the purpose of reimbursement for services provided by the physician.

RECORDING DIAGNOSES AND PROCEDURES

diagnosis *a physician's opinion of the nature of an illness or injury.*

procedures *services performed by a provider.*

When the patient sees the physician, the complaint(s) and symptom(s) are entered in the patient's medical record. The **diagnosis**, which is the physician's opinion of the nature of the patient's illness or injury, as well as the **procedures**—the services performed—are recorded. Medications prescribed are also listed.

Diagnoses are recorded not as narrative descriptions, such as carpal tunnel syndrome, but as codes, such as 354.0. The same is true for procedures. An electrocardiogram is not referred to as an electrocardiogram or an ECG, but as 93000. Coding is a way of translating a description of a condition into a shorter, standardized code. Standardization allows information to be shared among physicians, office personnel, insurance carriers, and so on, without losing its precise meaning. Diagnosis and procedure codes are very precise. Insurance carriers base much of their claim approval decisions on the information indicated by diagnosis and procedure codes. Thus, coding must only be done by someone in the medical office with specialized knowledge.

diagnosis code *a standardized value used to describe a patient's illness, signs, and symptoms.*

A patient's diagnosis is communicated to the insurance carrier as a **diagnosis code**, a code found in a reference text called the

FAMILY CARE CENTER PATIENT INFORMATION FORM
(PLEASE COMPLETE **ALL** INFORMATION)

PATIENT'S NAME _____ DATE OF BIRTH ___/___/___ SEX M❑ F❑ AGE_____

        Last Name   First Name   Middle Initial   M   D   Y

PATIENT'S STATUS   Single ❑   Married ❑   Widowed ❑   Divorced ❑   Separated ❑

PATIENT'S ADDRESS (No., Street) _____

                   City _____ State _____ ZIP Code_____

HOME TELEPHONE (_____) _____ SOCIAL SECURITY NUMBER _____ ____ _____

PATIENT'S RELATIONSHIP TO INSURED   Self ❑   Spouse ❑   Child ❑   Other ❑

ALLERGIES_____ REASON FOR VISIT _____

REFERRED BY _____

STUDENT STATUS   Full time ❑   Part time ❑   Non-student ❑

PATIENT'S OCCUPATION_____	SPOUSE'S OR PARENT'S NAME_____
EMPLOYMENT STATUS_____	OCCUPATION _____
EMPLOYER'S NAME _____	EMPLOYER'S NAME_____
BUSINESS ADDRESS _____	BUSINESS ADDRESS _____
City_____ State_____	City _____ State_____
ZIP Code _____	ZIP Code _____
BUSINESS TELEPHONE _____ (Include Area Code)	BUSINESS TELEPHONE_____ (Include Area Code)

PRIMARY INSURANCE PLAN			IS THERE A SECONDARY HEALTH BENEFIT PLAN?
PLAN NAME	PATIENT'S ID #		❑ YES ❑ NO *If yes, complete below.*
POLICYHOLDER'S NAME (Last Name, First Name, Middle Initial)			OTHER POLICYHOLDER'S NAME (Last Name, First Name, Middle Initial)
POLICYHOLDER'S ADDRESS (No. Street)			EMPLOYER'S NAME OR SCHOOL NAME
CITY	STATE	ZIP CODE	INSURANCE PLAN NAME OR PROGRAM NAME
% OF COVERAGE	TELEPHONE (INCLUDE AREA CODE) ( )		SECOND POLICY'S GROUP NUMBER AND I.D. NUMBER
POLICYHOLDER'S GROUP AND SOCIAL SECURITY NUMBER			
POLICYHOLDER'S DATE OF BIRTH SEX M❘ D❘ Y M❑ F❑			POLICYHOLDER'S DATE OF BIRTH SEX M❘ D❘ Y M❑ F❑

Regardless of any insurance coverage I/we may or may not have, it is my/our responsibility to pay the entire bill. In the event that this office needs to obtain legal assistance in collection of any unpaid balance, I/we agree to pay costs and attorney fees, as allowable by law, and acknowledge receipt of a photocopy of this agreement.

I/we authorize the release of the above patient's medical records for billing purposes.

_____   _____   _____
       Signature   Signature   Date

I/we authorize payment of medical benefits to the physician listed below.

_____   _____   _____
     Signature   Signature   Physician   Date

Figure 1-1 Sample patient information form.

International Classification of Diseases (ICD). Diagnosis codes provide insurance carriers with very specific information about the patient's specific illness(es), sign(s), and symptom(s). Errors in coding can delay the processing of claims and result in a reduced payment or the denial of a claim.

procedure code a standardized value that specifies which medical tests and procedures were performed.

Similarly, a **procedure code** is a standardized code that specifies which medical procedures and tests were performed. The most commonly used system of procedure codes is found in the *Physicians' Current Procedural Terminology*, Fourth Edition, also known as the *CPT*. The *CPT* was developed to provide a standardized system to use when describing diagnostic and therapeutic procedures.

superbill a form listing procedures relevant to the specialty of a medical office, used to indicate what procedures were performed.

After entering diagnostic and procedural information in the patient's medical record, the physician completes a **superbill**, also known as an encounter form (see Figure 1-2). The superbill lists procedures relevant to the particular specialty of the medical office and may also include a list of typical diagnoses. It may provide a place for office visit charges and payments. The information on superbills should be checked on an annual basis to be sure that all current diagnoses and procedures are listed.

BILLING PATIENTS AND FILING INSURANCE CLAIMS

During a typical day, dozens of patients visit the medical office. They have a variety of problems and needs, and they receive different services from the physician. When patients receive services from a medical practice, they either pay for services themselves or the charges are submitted to their insurance company or governmental agency for payment. To receive payment, most medical practices must complete or produce documents for insurance carriers and patients. One kind of document is an insurance claim form. Although some private insurance carriers have specialized claim forms for their policyholders, most forms ask for the same basic information. Fortunately, most insurance carriers also accept a universal claim form called the **Health Insurance Claim Form**, approved by the American Medical Association and the Health Care Financing Administration. This form is commonly known as the **HCFA-1500**, or the HCFA (pronounced "Hic-Fa") form. As illustrated in Figure 1-3 on page 8, this form is used for governmental health programs and many private plans.

Health Insurance Claim Form (HCFA-1500) a universal health insurance claim form used by governmental health programs and many private insurance carriers.

patient statement a document that informs the patient of the amount owed to the medical practice.

Sometimes charges are not covered by an insurance carrier; these charges must be billed to the patient. The **patient statement** informs the patient of the amount owed for a specific visit. The patient statement lists all services performed along with the associated charges. Most medical practices have a regular schedule, perhaps daily or weekly, for submitting claims to insurance carriers. For example, some practices bill half the patients on the fifteenth of the month and the other half on the thirtieth.

Family Care Center

285 Stephenson Boulevard
Stephenson, OH 60089
(614)555-0000

Date: 12/8/03   Name _____

Chart Number_____   Physician _____

01	patient payment, cash	85651	erythrocyte sedimentation rate--non-auto
02	patient payment, check	86403	strep test, quick
03	insurance carrier payment	86585	tuberculosis, tine test
04	insurance company adjustment	86588	direct streptococcus screen
05	adjustment, patient	87072	culture by commercial kit, nonurine...
06	OhioCare HMO Charge - $10	87076	bacterial culture, anerobic, with GC...
07	OhioCare HMO Charge - $15	87086	urine culture and colony count
12011	simple suture--face--local anes.	90703	tetanus injection
29125	application of short arm splint; static	90782	injection with material, subcutaneous or
29425	application of short leg cast, walking	92516	facial nerve function studies
45378	colonoscopy--diagnostic	93000	Electrocardiogram--ECG with interpret...
45380	colonoscopy--with biopsy	93015	Treadmill stress test, with physician...
50390	aspiration of renal cyst by needle	96900	ultraviolet light treatment
71010	chest x-ray, single view, frontal	99070	supplies and materials provided
71020	chest x-ray, two views, frontal & lat...	99201	OF--new patient, problem focused
71030	chest x-ray, complete, four views	99202	OF--new patient, expanded
73070	elbow x-ray, AP and lateral views	99203	OF--new patient, detailed history and...
73090	forearm x-ray, AP and lateral views	99204	OF--new patient, comprehensive history..
73100	wrist x-ray, AP and lateral views	99205	OF--new patient, comprehensive history..
73510	hip x-ray, complete, two views	99211	OF--established patient, minimal
73600	ankle x-ray, AP and lateral views	99212	OF--established patient, problem focused
80019	19 clinical chemistry tests	99213	OF--established patient, expanded
80061	lipid panel	99214	OF--established patient, detailed...
82270	blood screening, occult; feces	99215	OF--established patient, comprehensive..
82947	glucose screening--quantitative	99394	established patient, adolescent, per...
82951	glucose tolerance test, three specimens	99396	established patient, 40-64 years, per...
83718	HDL cholesterol		
84478	triglycerides test		
85007	manual differential WBC		
85022	hemogram, automated, and manual...		

Payments _____   Remarks _____

Diagnosis _____   _____

Figure 1-2 *Sample superbill.*

APPROVED OMB-0938-0008

CARRIER →

| | PICA | | | | HEALTH INSURANCE CLAIM FORM | | PICA | | |

HEALTH INSURANCE CLAIM FORM

1. MEDICARE	MEDICAID	CHAMPUS	CHAMPVA	GROUP HEALTH PLAN	FECA BLK LUNG	OTHER	1a. INSURED'S I.D. NUMBER (FOR PROGRAM IN ITEM 1)
☐ (Medicare #)	☐ (Medicaid #)	☐ (Sponsor's SSN)	☐ (VA File #)	☐ (SSN or ID)	☐ (SSN)	☐ (ID)	

2. PATIENT'S NAME (Last Name, First Name, Middle Initial)

3. PATIENT'S BIRTH DATE MM ¦ DD ¦ YY   SEX M ☐ F ☐

4. INSURED'S NAME (Last Name, First Name, Middle Initial)

5. PATIENT'S ADDRESS (No., Street)

6. PATIENT RELATIONSHIP TO INSURED Self ☐ Spouse ☐ Child ☐ Other ☐

7. INSURED'S ADDRESS (No., Street)

CITY   STATE

8. PATIENT STATUS Single ☐ Married ☐ Other ☐

CITY   STATE

ZIP CODE   TELEPHONE (Include Area Code) ( )

Employed ☐ Full-Time Student ☐ Part-Time Student ☐

ZIP CODE   TELEPHONE (INCLUDE AREA CODE) ( )

9. OTHER INSURED'S NAME (Last Name, First Name, Middle Initial)

10. IS PATIENT'S CONDITION RELATED TO:

11. INSURED'S POLICY GROUP OR FECA NUMBER

a. OTHER INSURED'S POLICY OR GROUP NUMBER

a. EMPLOYMENT? (CURRENT OR PREVIOUS) ☐ YES ☐ NO

a. INSURED'S DATE OF BIRTH MM ¦ DD ¦ YY   SEX M ☐ F ☐

b. OTHER INSURED'S DATE OF BIRTH MM ¦ DD ¦ YY   SEX M ☐ F ☐

b. AUTO ACCIDENT? PLACE (State) ☐ YES ☐ NO

b. EMPLOYER'S NAME OR SCHOOL NAME

c. EMPLOYER'S NAME OR SCHOOL NAME

c. OTHER ACCIDENT? ☐ YES ☐ NO

c. INSURANCE PLAN NAME OR PROGRAM NAME

d. INSURANCE PLAN NAME OR PROGRAM NAME

10d. RESERVED FOR LOCAL USE

d. IS THERE ANOTHER HEALTH BENEFIT PLAN? ☐ YES ☐ NO **If yes,** return to and complete item 9 a-d.

READ BACK OF FORM BEFORE COMPLETING & SIGNING THIS FORM.

12. PATIENT'S OR AUTHORIZED PERSON'S SIGNATURE I authorize the release of any medical or other information necessary to process this claim. I also request payment of government benefits either to myself or to the party who accepts assignment below.

SIGNED _____ DATE _____

13. INSURED'S OR AUTHORIZED PERSON'S SIGNATURE I authorize payment of medical benefits to the undersigned physician or supplier for services described below.

SIGNED _____

14. DATE OF CURRENT: MM ¦ DD ¦ YY ◄ ILLNESS (First symptom) OR INJURY (Accident) OR PREGNANCY (LMP)

15. IF PATIENT HAS HAD SAME OR SIMILAR ILLNESS, GIVE FIRST DATE MM ¦ DD ¦ YY

16. DATES PATIENT UNABLE TO WORK IN CURRENT OCCUPATION FROM MM ¦ DD ¦ YY TO MM ¦ DD ¦ YY

17. NAME OF REFERRING PHYSICIAN OR OTHER SOURCE

17a. I.D. NUMBER OF REFERRING PHYSICIAN

18. HOSPITALIZATION DATES RELATED TO CURRENT SERVICES FROM MM ¦ DD ¦ YY TO MM ¦ DD ¦ YY

19. RESERVED FOR LOCAL USE

20. OUTSIDE LAB? ☐ YES ☐ NO $ CHARGES

21. DIAGNOSIS OR NATURE OF ILLNESS OR INJURY. (RELATE ITEMS 1,2,3, OR 4 TO ITEM 24E BY LINE)

1. L___ . __   3. L___ . __
2. L___ . __   4. L___ . __

22. MEDICAID RESUBMISSION CODE   ORIGINAL REF. NO.

23. PRIOR AUTHORIZATION NUMBER

24. A DATE(S) OF SERVICE		B Place of Service	C Type of Service	D PROCEDURES, SERVICES, OR SUPPLIES (Explain Unusual Circumstances)		E DIAGNOSIS CODE	F $ CHARGES	G DAYS OR UNITS	H EPSDT Family Plan	I EMG	J COB	K RESERVED FOR LOCAL USE
From MM DD YY	To MM DD YY			CPT/HCPCS	MODIFIER							
1												
2												
3												
4												
5												
6												

25. FEDERAL TAX I.D. NUMBER SSN ☐ EIN ☐

26. PATIENT'S ACCOUNT NO.

27. ACCEPT ASSIGNMENT? (For govt. claims, see back) ☐ YES ☐ NO

28. TOTAL CHARGE $

29. AMOUNT PAID $

30. BALANCE DUE $

31. SIGNATURE OF PHYSICIAN OR SUPPLIER INCLUDING DEGREES OR CREDENTIALS (I certify that the statements on the reverse apply to this bill and are made a part thereof.)

SIGNED _____ DATE _____

32. NAME AND ADDRESS OF FACILITY WHERE SERVICES WERE RENDERED (if other than home or office)

33. PHYSICIAN'S OR SUPPLIER'S NAME, ADDRESS, ZIP CODE & TELEPHONE NO.

PIN#   GRP#

(APPROVED BY AMA COUNCIL ON MEDICAL SERVICE 8/88)   **PLEASE PRINT OR TYPE**

FORM HCFA-1500 (12-90)
FORM OWCP-1500   FORM RRB-1500

PATIENT AND INSURED INFORMATION →

PHYSICIAN OR SUPPLIER INFORMATION →

Figure 1-3 Health Insurance Claim Form (HCFA-1500).

Overview of Medical Insurance

There is a wide variety of medical insurance plans in the United States. Many people are covered by a group policy, often through their employer. Other people, such as those who are self-employed, have individual plans. Insurance coverage may be supplied by a private company, such as Aetna, or it can be a governmental plan. Some of the most common governmental plans in effect in the United States are:

◆ ✓**CHAMPUS**　The Civilian Health and Medical Program of the Uniformed Services covers medical expenses for dependents of active-duty members of the uniformed services and for retired military personnel. It also covers dependents of military personnel who were killed while on active duty.

◆ ✓**CHAMPVA**　The Civilian Health and Medical Program of the Veterans Administration is for veterans with permanent service-related disabilities and their dependents. It also covers surviving spouses and dependent children of veterans who died from service-related disabilities.

◆ ✓**Medicare**　Medicare is a federal health plan that covers persons aged 65 and over, people with disabilities, and dependent widows.

◆ ✓**Medicaid**　People with low incomes who cannot afford medical care are covered by Medicaid, which is cosponsored by federal and state governments. Qualifications and benefits vary by state.

◆ ✓**Workers' Compensation**　People with job-related illnesses or injuries are covered under workers' compensation insurance. Workers' compensation benefits vary according to state law.

Whether private company or governmental program, the insurance carrier is called a **third-party payer**. The primary relationship is between the physician and the patient. The insurance carrier is the third party.

Different types of insurance plans can be purchased. In an **indemnity plan**, policyholders are paid back for costs they experience when they pay for health care due to illnesses and accidents. Under an indemnity plan, the **schedule of benefits** in the policy lists the services that are covered and the amounts that are paid. The benefit may be for all or part of the charges. For example, the schedule of benefits may indicate that 80 percent of charges for surgery performed in a hospital are covered while the policyholder is responsible for paying the other 20 percent. This is known as **coinsurance**.

Another type of insurance system is managed care. **Managed care** was introduced in the mid-1980s as a way of supervising health care to be sure patients get the necessary care in the most appropriate, cost-effective setting. A managed care company is responsible for both the financing and the delivery of health care to its policyholders. The

third-party payer a term used to describe an insurance carrier in the context of the physician's and the patient's relationship.

indemnity plan an insurance plan in which policyholders are reimbursed for health care costs.

schedule of benefits in an insurance policy, a listing of services covered and the amount of coverage.

coinsurance a type of insurance plan in which the patient is responsible for a percentage of the charges.

managed care a type of insurance in which the insurance carrier is responsible for the financing and the delivery of health care.

company signs up providers who agree to supply services for a fixed fee. The providers do not set the fees. Instead, they are set by the company or governmental agency that has a contract with the providers. One common type of managed care system is a **health maintenance organization (HMO)**. In an HMO, patients pay fixed rates at regular intervals, such as monthly. In some HMOs, they also pay a **copayment**—a small fixed fee, such as $10, at the time of the office visit. In HMOs patients must choose from a specific group of physicians and hospitals for their medical care.

Processing Claims

For an insurance carrier to pay a claim, certain information about the patient must be shared. For example, the insurance carrier needs to know the physician's assessment of the patient's condition—the patient's diagnosis—and the procedures the physician performed while the patient was in the office. The date of the visit and the location of the visit (such as physician's office or hospital) also must be recorded. The insurance carrier also requires basic information about the physician providing the treatment, including the provider's name and/or provider identification number.

The information needed to create a claim is found on the patient information form and the superbill. Some insurance claims are mailed to insurance carriers on paper forms. Other claims are submitted electronically by transferring information from a computer in the provider's office to a computer at the insurance company.

When the claim is received by the insurance carrier, it is reviewed and processed. If the patient's insurance is an indemnity plan, the insurance company compares the fees to the schedule of benefits in the patient's policy and determines the amount of benefit to be paid. If the patient's insurance coverage is a managed care plan, the insurance company pays a contracted fee to the provider and the patient pays a copayment directly to the provider.

REVIEWING AND RECORDING PAYMENTS

After the amount of the benefit is determined, the insurance carrier issues a payment. At the same time, it issues an **explanation of benefits (EOB)** or remittance advice. An EOB indicates how the amount of benefit was determined (see Figure 1-4). The insurance company may send the payment to the physician or to the policyholder.

When the EOB arrives at the physician's office, it is reviewed for accuracy. If an error is found, a request for a review of the claim must be filed with the carrier. If a check is enclosed, the amount of the payment from the insurance carrier is recorded. The patient is billed for any outstanding balance.

CUSTOMER'S EXPLANATION OF BENEFITS

1324   0664402

THIS IS NOT A BILL. RETAIN FOR YOUR RECORDS.

CUSTOMER'S NAME: SUSAN BILTON
ID NUMBER: 140385526
PATIENT'S NAME: SUSAN BILTON

COVERAGE: BCBS OF NJ

CONSUMER DIVISION

CLAIM NUMBER: 7970920006160000
CLAIM RECEIVED: 04/02/99
CLAIM FINALIZED: 04/08/99
CHECK NUMBER: 0005890315

MEDICAL SURGICAL/MAJOR MEDICAL CLAIM SUMMARY

CHARGES FOR THIS CLAIM	$ 1,224.00
AMOUNT OF CUSTOMER BALANCE REMAINING	$ 367.20
BENEFITS PAID TO SUSAN BILTON	$ 856.80

DO NOT SUBMIT A SEPARATE MAJOR MEDICAL CLAIM FORM
THIS CLAIM HAS BEEN PROCESSED UNDER YOUR MEDICAL-SURGICAL AND MAJOR MEDICAL CONTRACTS

PATIENT'S NAME: SUSAN BILTON   IDENTIFICATION NUMBER: 140385526   CLAIM NUMBER: 7970920006160000

PROVIDER NAME		1	2	3	4	5	6	7	8	9
TYPE OF SERVICE -	DATE OF SERVICE	CHARGE	OTHER INS	NOT COVERED	ELIGIBLE	DEDUC-	COINS/	BENEFIT	CUSTOMER	MSG
PLACE OF SERVICE	FROM TO	AMOUNT	PAYMENT	AMOUNT	AMOUNT	TIBLE	CO-PAY	AMOUNT	BALANCE	CODES
ANESTHESIA CONSLTNTS CENTRL JERSEY										
ANESTHESIA-INPATIENT 03/13/99 03/13/99		1224.00			1224.00		367.20	856.80		
MAJOR MEDICAL		1224.00						0.00	367.20	
THIS IS NOT A BILL										
TOTALS		1224.00			1224.00		367.20	856.80	367.20	
MESSAGES										

CRP02B (1-97)

* SUSAN HAS SATISFIED $1,000.00 OF HER DEDUCTIBLE FOR THE PERIOD 01-01-99 TO 12-31-99. (OO55)

Figure 1-4 Sample explanation of benefits statement.

CHAPTER REVIEW

USING TERMINOLOGY

Match the terms on the left with the definitions on the right.

_____ **1.** coinsurance

_T_ **2.** copayment

_____ **3.** diagnosis

_____ **4.** diagnosis code

_a_ **5.** explanation of benefits (EOB)

_____ **6.** health maintenance organization (HMO)

_____ **7.** indemnity plan

_____ **8.** insurance carrier

_b_ **9.** Health Insurance Claim Form (HCFA-1500)

_____ **10.** managed care

_c_ **11.** patient information form

_____ **12.** patient statement

_____ **13.** policyholder

_____ **14.** premiums

_____ **15.** procedure code

a. A document from an insurance carrier that lists the amount of a benefit and explains how it was determined.

b. A universal health insurance claim form used by governmental health programs and many private insurance carriers.

c. A document that contains personal, employment, and medical insurance information about a patient.

d. A document that informs the patient of the amount owed to the medical practice.

e. A form listing procedures relevant to the specialty of a medical office, used to indicate what procedures were performed.

f. In an insurance policy, a listing of services covered and the amount of coverage.

g. A term used to describe an insurance carrier in the context of the physician's and the patient's relationship.

h. Services performed by a provider.

i. An individual who has contracted with an insurance company for coverage.

j. Payments made to an insurance carrier by a policyholder for coverage.

k. A type of insurance in which the carrier is responsible for the financing and the delivery of health care.

l. A physician's opinion of the nature of an illness or injury.

m. A standardized value used to describe a patient's illness, signs, and symptoms.

n. An insurance plan in which policyholders are reimbursed for health care costs.

o. A type of insurance plan in which the patient is responsible for a percentage of the charges.

_____ **16.** procedures

_____ **17.** providers

_____ **18.** schedule of benefits

_____ **19.** superbill

_____ **20.** third-party payer

p. A standardized value that specifies which medical tests and procedures were performed.

q. Physicians, hospitals, and other medical staff who provide medical services.

r. A company that provides insurance coverage to individuals and/or groups.

s. A type of managed care system in which patients pay fixed rates at regular intervals.

t. A small fixed fee paid by the patient at the time of an office visit.

CHECKING YOUR UNDERSTANDING

Write "T" or "F" in the blank to indicate whether you think the statement is true or false.

_____ **21.** Many patient information forms contain a place for the patient to sign to authorize an insurance carrier to send payments directly to a provider.

_____ **22.** Insurance carriers look closely at procedure and diagnosis codes when making claim approval decisions.

_____ **23.** Coinsurance refers to a small fixed fee that must be paid by the patient at the time of an office visit.

_____ **24.** To receive payment for services, most medical offices must produce two documents—a patient statement and an insurance claim form.

Answer the question below in the space provided.

25. List the five basic categories of administrative tasks in a medical office.

_____

_____

_____

_____

_____

CHAPTER REVIEW

Choose the best answer.

_____ **26.** A patient information form contains information such as name, address, employer, and:
  a. diagnosis code
  b. insurance coverage information
  c. charges for procedures performed

_____ **27.** A health maintenance organization (HMO) is one example of a(n):
  a. indemnity plan
  b. governmental plan
  c. managed care plan

_____ **28.** In a managed care plan, payments are made:
  a. to the patient at the time of the office visit
  b. to the patient after a claim has been filed
  c. to the provider

_____ **29.** The most commonly used system of procedure codes is found in the:
  a. *CPT*
  b. *ICD*
  c. HCFA-1500

_____ **30.** Information about a patient's medical procedures that is needed to create an insurance claim is found on the:
  a. explanation of benefits
  b. patient statement
  c. superbill

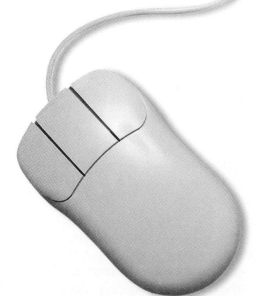

CHAPTER 2

The Role of Computers in the Medical Office

OBJECTIVES

In this chapter, you will learn:

◆ How medical offices use computers to accomplish daily administrative tasks.

◆ The advantages that computers offer over traditional paper methods in the medical practice.

◆ The common applications of computer systems in the medical office, including scheduling, accounting, filing electronic media claims, word processing, and using the Internet.

KEY TERMS

audit/edit report
clearinghouse
computer literacy
database
electronic funds transfer (EFT)
electronic media claim (EMC)

electronic remittance advice (ERA)
Internet
modem
network
transaction information
walkout receipt

INTRODUCTION TO THE ROLE OF COMPUTERS IN THE MEDICAL OFFICE

computer literacy the
knowledge of how to use
computers to perform work.

In the past, most of the administrative work carried out in the medical office involved paper. Appointments were recorded in scheduling books, insurance claims were printed on paper forms, physician's schedules were often prepared with handwritten notes, and so on. All this paper had to be filed and stored. Powerful, inexpensive computer technology introduced in the 1980s paved the way for the use of computers in the medical office. Today, most medical offices have at least one computer and use it regularly to produce insurance claims, create reports on the office's finances, schedule appointments, handle payroll, prepare letters and memos, and so on. **Computer literacy,** the knowledge of how to use computers to perform desired work, is an increasingly important ability required of medical office employees.

The tasks discussed in Chapter 1 (see Table 2-1) are performed on a regular basis in most medical offices. In each instance, the task can be completed more efficiently with the use of a specialized computer application.

Table 2-1   Computer Applications of Medical Office Administrative Tasks

Task	Computer Application
Scheduling appointments.	Appointment scheduled electronically.
Gathering and recording patient information.	Data entered into computer database.
Recording diagnoses and procedures.	Data entered into computer database.
Billing patients and filing insurance claims.	Patient statements and insurance claims generated by computer; claims transmitted electronically.
Reviewing and recording payment.	Data entered into computer database; claim refiled or patient statement generated.

To understand the role that computers play in today's medical office, consider the following typical day in a computerized medical office. At the beginning of each day, the computer is used to print a listing of all appointments for that day for each physician in the office (see Figure 2-1). New appointments are booked during the day using an electronic scheduling program. New/revised data on patient information forms, such as patients' addresses, insurance plans, allergies, and so on, are entered into the computer database. As

Appointments:Yan, Katherine   **Friday - November 21, 2003**

Time	Name	Phone	Length	Message
8:00a	Fitzwilliams, John	(614)002-1111	30	
8:15a	_____	_____		_____
8:30a	_____	_____		_____
8:45a	Ramos, Maritza	(614)315-2233	45	
9:00a	_____	_____		_____
9:15a	_____	_____		_____
9:30a	_____	_____		_____
9:45a	Staff Meeting		15	
10:00a	Staff Meeting		15	
10:15a	Staff Meeting		15	
10:30a	Staff Meeting		15	
10:45a	Staff Meeting		15	
11:00a	_____	_____		
11:15a	Smolowski, James	(614)077-2249	15	
11:30a	Bell, Samuel	(614)030-1111	15	
11:45a	Bell, Sarina	(614)030-1111	15	
12:00n	Lunch		15	
12:15n	Lunch		15	
12:30n	Lunch		15	
12:45n	Lunch		15	
1:00p	Gardiner, John	(614)726-9898	60	
1:15p	_____	_____		_____
1:30p	_____	_____		_____
1:45p	_____	_____		_____
2:00p	_____	_____		_____
2:15p	Patterson, Leila	(614)666-0099	30	
2:30p	_____	_____		_____
2:45p	Jones, Elizabeth	(614)123-5555	30	
3:00p	_____	_____		_____
3:15p	_____	_____		_____
3:30p	Smith, Sarabeth	(614)822-0000	45	
3:45p	_____	_____		_____
4:00p	_____	_____		_____
4:15p	_____	_____		_____
4:30p	Wong, Jo	(614)029-7777	15	
4:45p	_____	_____		_____

Printed at 11/22/03 10:02:00 AM   Page 1

Figure 2-1 *Sample computerized appointment schedule for a physician (MediSoft).*

the physicians see patients, diagnoses and procedures are recorded on computer-generated superbills. When an office visit is completed, information from the superbill is entered into the computerized billing program. The computer can then be used to print a **walkout receipt** for the patient (see Figure 2-2) and later to create and print an insurance claim. Instead of printing and mailing insurance claim forms, the medical office assistant may use the computer to electronically transmit claims to the insurance carriers for payment. When a payment is received, it is recorded in the computer and the patient is billed for any remaining balance. At the end of the day, reports are printed showing the daily activity of the practice—the number of patient visits, the diagnosis and procedure codes used, the fees charged, and the payments received.

walkout receipt *a document listing charges and payments that is given to a patient after an office visit.*

ADVANTAGES OF COMPUTERS

There are a number of advantages to using computers for tasks in the medical office. Most computerized medical office systems are structured as a collection of related facts called a **database**. A medical office computer database stores information about providers, patients, insurance carriers, procedure codes, diagnoses, charges, and payments. There are several advantages to storing information in a computer database rather than in paper files. With a computer database, all the information is located in one place. Pieces of paper and forms are not located in different file cabinets in the office; they are all stored on one computer system.

database *a collection of related facts.*

In addition, computer data can be used by more than one person at a time. If an office has more than one computer, the computers can be linked together in a **network,** which allows them to share files in the central database. In an office without a computer database, it is difficult for someone to update a document if another person is working on it.

network *a series of computers that are linked together, allowing them to share files.*

Another advantage of computer databases is the simplicity of conducting a search for information. Instead of having to look in different file cabinets and folders, a search can be conducted by just entering a few keystrokes. In a very short time, the information is retrieved and displayed on the computer screen.

The most important advantage that computer databases offer over manual filing systems is the ability to link related pieces of information to process insurance claim forms. When preparing patients' claims, the computer selects information from its databases to create an electronic file of the information needed to complete the claim forms. Those claim forms can then be printed or transmitted electronically.

Family Care Center
285 Stephenson Boulevard
Stephenson, OH 60089
(614)555-0000

11/22/03

Patient: **Paul Ramos**
39 Locust Avenue
Stephenson, OH 60089

Diagnosis: 1. 706.1
2.
3.
4.

Account Number: RAMOSPA0
Case #: 13

Instructions: Complete the patient information portion of your own insurance claim form. Attach this bill, signed and dated, and all other bills pertaining to the claim. If you have a deductible policy, hold your claim forms until you have met your deductible. Mail directly to your insurance carrier.

Date	Description	Procedure	Modify	DX	Units	Charge
9/17/02	OF--new patient focused	99201		1	1	140.00
9/17/02	ultraviolet light treatment	96900		1	1	23.50

Provider Information
Provider Name:	John Rudner MD
License:	84701
Insurance PIN:	
SSN or EIN:	339-67-5000

Total Charges:	163.50
Total Credits:	0.00
Total Due This Visit:	$ 163.50
Total Balance Due:	$ 163.50

Assign and Release: I hereby authorize payment of medical benefits to this physician for the services described above. I also authorize the release of any information necessary to process this claim.

Patient Signature: _____   Date: _____

Figure 2-2 Sample walkout receipt (MediSoft).

Bringing computers into the medical office has greatly increased productivity, primarily because computers are much more efficient at processing large amounts of data than human beings. Tasks that would take minutes for a human to complete can be done by the computer in a matter of seconds. For example, suppose a medical practice has multiple providers and hundreds of patients. The phone rings, and a patient would like to know the amount owed on an account. With a computerized billing program in place, the medical office assistant might simply key the first few letters of the patient's last name into the computer, causing the patient's account to appear on the screen. The outstanding balance then could be communicated to the patient.

In another example, suppose the wrong diagnosis code has been written on an insurance claim form, and the claim has been rejected by the insurance carrier. To resubmit the claim without the use of a computer might require the entire form to be completed again by hand. However, if the medical office used a computerized billing program, the error could be corrected in seconds and a new form either printed, or submitted electronically.

Computers not only make the medical office more efficient, they also reduce errors. Working with a computer system, there is less chance for error, in part because information is entered once and then used over and over again. Once information is entered, provided it is entered correctly the first time, it will be correct every time it is used. For example, information such as the patient's address and insurance policy number is entered in the computer once. The computer stores the information and when the information is needed to fill out a claim form, the computer locates it and uses it to complete the task, such as printing a completed claim form. The next time a claim form needs to be completed, the computer goes through the same process, using the same information. Without a computer, someone would have to key all the information on an insurance form each time a claim was being submitted for the patient. Not only does this consume more time, but it introduces the possibility for error every time the information has to be rekeyed.

Computerized billing systems also make it easier to focus on checking that procedure and diagnosis codes are related in the correct way. This is essential if insurance claims are to be paid in a timely manner. If a procedure code does not relate to the diagnosis code, the claim will be rejected, even though the procedure may be one that is covered under the patient's policy. For example, suppose a patient sees the doctor and is diagnosed with acute sinusitis. The physician ordered X rays of the patient's sinus cavities to arrive at this diagnosis. However, the procedure code was incorrectly entered as a forearm X ray. The insurance company will not pay the claim, because the procedure is not related to the diagnosis.

While computers do increase the efficiency of the medical office and reduce errors, computers are not more accurate than the individual entering the data. If human errors occur while entering the information, the data coming out of the computer will be incorrect. Computers are very precise and also very unforgiving. While the human brain knows flu is short for influenza, the computer does not know this and regards these as two distinct conditions. If a computer operator accidentally enters a name as "ORourke" instead of "O'Rourke," a human might know what is meant; the computer does not. It would probably respond with a message such as "No such patient exists in the database."

Most human errors occur during data entry, such as pressing the wrong key on the keyboard or because of the lack of computer literacy—not knowing how to use a program to accomplish the tasks. For this reason, proper training in data-entry techniques and computer programs is essential for medical office personnel who are working with computers.

SCHEDULING APPLICATIONS

Computers are often used to keep track of physicians' schedules. Appointments can easily be canceled, moved to a different day, and so on. Computers can also print a daily list of appointments for each provider in the practice. Recurring appointments can be booked for future dates, such as once a week for the next six weeks.

One of the major advantages of computerized scheduling is the ability to locate scheduled appointments easily. For example, suppose a patient calls to ask when his or her next appointment is scheduled. Instead of searching page by page in a paper schedule book, the medical office assistant enters the patient's name in a search box and the computer locates the appointment. Computer scheduling programs are also used to store information about time reserved for surgeries, seminars, lunches, days off, and so on.

ACCOUNTING APPLICATIONS

As with other businesses, medical offices keep track of accounts receivable, payments coming in from patients and insurance carriers; and accounts payable, amounts owed to suppliers and staff. Keeping accurate financial records is critical to the practice's survival. Not only are accurate records needed to meet financial obligations, but they are also required for tax-reporting purposes. And, as in any business, accurate financial reports let management know whether the medical office is profitable.

Computerized accounting programs perform the tasks that were accomplished manually in the past. Medical offices may use different computerized accounting systems to keep track of their finances, but all accounting systems require certain types of information:

♦ **Patient data**   Personal information about the patient, as well as information on the patient's insurance coverage, is extracted from the program's patient database.

♦ **Transaction data   Transaction information** is taken from the superbill and keyed into the computer program. It includes the date of the visit, diagnosis and procedure codes, lab work, medications prescribed, and payments.

transaction information data about an office visit taken from the superbill.

From these sources of information, patient statements are generated, insurance claims are created, and reports on the financial health of the practice are produced.

One of the major uses of computer technology in the medical office is in creating insurance claims. A computerized system automatically generates completed insurance forms. The forms can be printed or transmitted electronically. By comparison, if a manual system is used, the medical office assistant must first compile all the needed resources and then key all the data on the claim form. This process is longer, and more likely to create processing errors.

MediSoft for Windows, the computerized health care billing system used in this text, is one example of a computer program used in the medical office to process insurance claims. Processing information to create completed insurance claim forms is one of the main functions of programs such as MediSoft. Three major steps are followed to create insurance claims using MediSoft: (1) setting up the practice, (2) entering transaction information, and (3) creating and transmitting the completed insurance claim form.

SETTING UP THE PRACTICE

Before a medical practice opens its doors to patients, a lot of preparation must be done. Equipment, supplies, staff, and procedures all need to be readied. Similarly, before MediSoft is used to store information about patients and their visits, basic facts about the practice itself are entered. Often a computer consultant or an accountant helps set up MediSoft's records about the practice. Then the provider database is entered, including descriptions of each physician's office hours and facts about referring physicians and lab services. Finally, the insurance carrier database is entered. It contains information about the carriers that most patients use. Within MediSoft, each database is linked, or related, to each of the others by having at least one fact in common.

ENTERING TRANSACTION INFORMATION

When a patient visits a physician, information about the visit is collected on the patient information form and the superbill. After analyzing and checking the data, the medical office assistant enters each element in the computer program. A new record must be created for a new patient, and established patients' information may need to be updated. Next, the appropriate insurance carrier for the visit is selected. Then, the purposes of the visit, the diagnosis codes, and the procedure codes are entered with the appropriate charges.

CREATING THE INSURANCE CLAIM FORM

When all transaction information has been entered and checked, the medical office assistant issues the command to MediSoft to create an insurance claim form. The format for the claim—either the HCFA-1500 or a specialized claim form—is also designated. MediSoft then organizes the necessary databases and selects the data from each database as needed to produce a complete claim form. The program follows the instructions to print or transmit the form electronically to the designated receiver.

ELECTRONIC MEDIA CLAIMS

An **electronic media claim (EMC)** is an insurance claim that is sent by a computer over a telephone line using a **modem**. Electronic claim filing has several advantages. It is faster to file and process claims electronically than to fill out and process paper forms, and it requires fewer staff members. In addition, it costs less to file electronically; the costs of paper forms, envelopes, and postage are much higher than the costs of transmission over phone lines. Also, the chance for error or omission is reduced because information is entered once, not twice. In the case of paper forms, information also has to be entered into the insurance company's computer when the forms arrive by mail.

electronic media claim (EMC) an insurance claim that is sent by a computer over a telephone line using a modem.

modem an electronic device that enables information to be sent from one computer to another over telephone lines.

Usually, EMCs are paid faster than paper claims. For example, Medicare pays electronic claims in about half the time it takes for paper claims to be paid. Another advantage for the provider of submitting an EMC is **electronic funds transfer (EFT)**. This capability, which is an optional part of most EMC processing systems, allows for payments to be deposited directly into the provider's bank account. Many carrier's systems are also set up to provide **electronic remittance advice (ERA)**. An ERA is an electronic explanation of benefits sent to the provider. (A paper EOB is mailed to the patient.) An ERA is much faster than a mailed EOB, since the information is transmitted directly to the provider's computer by modem. Questions can thus be resolved faster, too, improving the provider's receipt of payment.

electronic funds transfer (EFT) a system that transfers money electronically from one account to another.

electronic remittance advice (ERA) an electronic explanation of benefits sent to the provider's computer by modem.

Problems with EMCs usually result when transmission failures occur due to power outages. Transmission problems may also result from the breakdown of computer equipment. In these cases, the remedy is to retransmit missing claims after the problem is solved.

Electronic media claims can be sent directly to an insurance carrier, or they can be sent to a clearinghouse. A **clearinghouse** is a service bureau that collects electronic insurance claims from many different medical practices and forwards the claims to the appropriate insurance carriers (see Figure 2-3). Some insurance carriers who receive insurance claims electronically require information to be formatted in a certain way. Clearinghouses translate claim data to fit the setup

clearinghouse a service bureau that collects electronic insurance claims and forwards them to the appropriate insurance carrier.

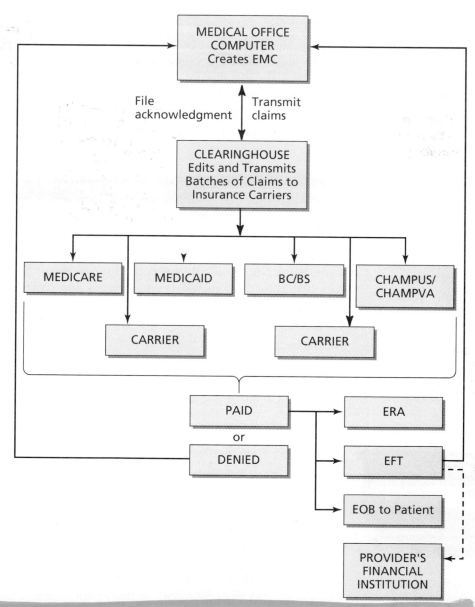

Figure 2-3 Example of EMC flow using a clearinghouse (courtesy of The Computer Place/MediSoft).

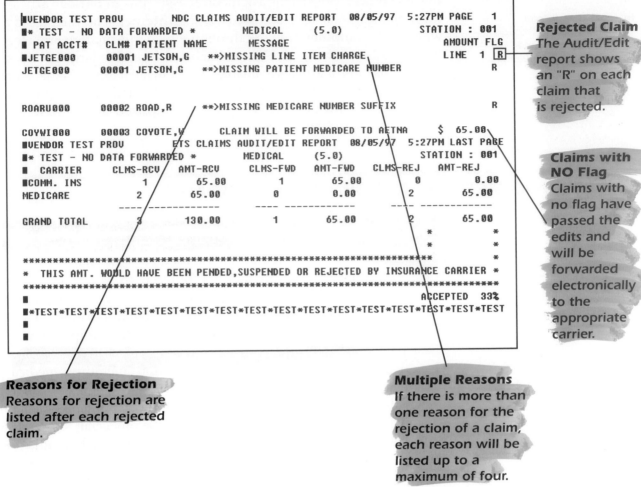

Rejected Claim The Audit/Edit report shows an "R" on each claim that is rejected.

Claims with NO Flag Claims with no flag have passed the edits and will be forwarded electronically to the appropriate carrier.

Reasons for Rejection Reasons for rejection are listed after each rejected claim.

Multiple Reasons If there is more than one reason for the rejection of a claim, each reason will be listed up to a maximum of four.

Figure 2-4 Sample audit/edit report.

of each carrier's claims processing department. Because of this factor, many medical practices choose to use a clearinghouse instead of transmitting claims directly to insurance carriers.

When a clearinghouse receives claims, it checks to see that all necessary information is included. An **audit/edit report** is used to communicate problems to the medical office that need to be corrected (see Figure 2-4). This reduces the number of claim rejections by insurance carriers and speeds the processing and payment of claims.

audit/edit report a report from a clearinghouse that lists errors that need to be corrected before a claim can be submitted to the insurance carrier.

WORD PROCESSING AND INTERNET APPLICATIONS

As with other businesses, medical offices use computers to produce written correspondence, reports, forms, and other documents. Computers are also used in the transcription of physician's notes about patients. Most word processing software includes a feature that checks spelling and grammar. While these features are useful, computerized spell-check programs do not eliminate the need for careful review by office personnel.

Internet *a worldwide computer network through which information and electronic mail is exchanged.*

In some offices, physicians ask medical assistants to retrieve articles from medical databases accessed via the **Internet**. The Internet is a worldwide computer network through which information and electronic mail is exchanged. Online databases resemble large libraries, with thousands of articles available. In a field such as medicine, with new treatments being discovered on an almost daily basis, access to timely data is invaluable. Using a computerized search, relevant articles can be located quickly.

ELECTRONIC MEDICAL RECORD APPLICATIONS

Systems are being developed that allow physicians' clinical notes on a patient's condition to be entered into a computer using a variety of technologies. Once clinical information is entered into the computer, it can be transmitted to another computer with just a few commands. This can be especially helpful in emergency situations. For example, suppose a patient had coronary bypass surgery eight weeks ago and today is admitted to the hospital complaining of chest pain. The computer at the physician's office could transmit clinical information on the patient's condition, including medications currently taken, and so on, to a computer at the hospital. The information would be available in seconds. Results of tests, such as electrocardiograms, could also be sent from the physician's computer to the hospital's computer for review. In a case such as this, in which time is critical, the computer can be another piece of lifesaving equipment. However, it may be years before electronic medical records systems are in wide use.

Storing patient records on the computer also brings up the issue of computer security and the confidentiality of patient records. Everyone working in a medical office is charged with the responsibility of maintaining patient confidentiality. Many states have laws that protect the patient's privacy. If the patient's medical record is stored on the computer, who should have access to that data? How will the data be safeguarded so it does not end up where it does not belong? In response to questions such as these, some organizations are developing guidelines for increased computer security. As one security measure, many medical offices assign passwords to individuals who have access to computer files, thereby limiting access to data stored on the computer.

CHAPTER REVIEW

USING TERMINOLOGY

Match the terms on the left with the definitions on the right.

_____ 1. audit/edit report

_____ 2. clearinghouse

_____ 3. computer literacy

_____ 4. database

_____ 5. electronic funds transfer (EFT)

_____ 6. electronic media claim (EMC)

_____ 7. electronic remittance advice (ERA)

_____ 8. Internet

_____ 9. modem

_____ 10. network

_____ 11. transaction information

_____ 12. walkout receipt

a. A series of computers that are linked together, allowing them to share files.

b. An insurance claim that is sent by a computer over a telephone line using a modem.

c. A system that transfers money electronically from one account to another.

d. The knowledge of how to use computers to perform work.

e. A worldwide computer network through which information and electronic mail is exchanged.

f. A service bureau that collects electronic insurance claims and forwards them to the appropriate insurance carrier.

g. An electronic explanation of benefits sent to the provider's computer by modem.

h. An electronic device that enables information to be sent from one computer to another over telephone lines.

i. A report from a clearinghouse that lists errors that need to be corrected before a claim can be submitted to the insurance carrier.

j. A document listing charges and payments that is given to a patient after an office visit.

k. A collection of related facts.

l. Data about an office visit taken from the superbill.

CHECKING YOUR UNDERSTANDING

Write "T" or "F" in the blank to indicate whether you think the statement is true or false.

_____ **13.** Computerized scheduling makes it easier to reschedule appointments in a medical office.

_____ **14.** Online databases store personal information on patient diagnoses.

_____ **15.** Many states have laws that protect the privacy of a patient's medical records.

_____ **16.** Electronic media claims are usually paid more quickly than claims submitted on paper forms.

Answer the questions below in the space provided.

17. List two advantages of using computers for tasks in the medical office.

_____

_____

18. Explain the advantage of electronic medical records over traditional paper records in an emergency situation.

_____

_____

Choose the best answer.

_____ **19.** Electronic remittance advice (ERA) is:
   a. the electronic transfer of funds from one bank account to another
   b. a report from a clearinghouse listing any errors in a claim
   c. an electronic explanation of benefits

_____ **20.** Systems that allow physicians' clinical notes to be stored in a computer are known as:
   a. Internet applications
   b. electronic medical records applications
   c. diagnosis coding applications

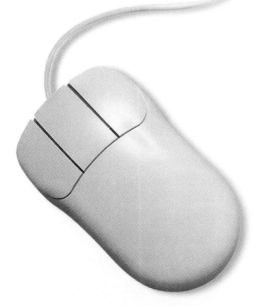

CHAPTER 3

An Overview of Microsoft Windows 95

OBJECTIVES

In this chapter, you will learn how to:

◆ Describe the basic components of a computer system.

◆ Start Windows 95.

◆ Identify the elements of the desktop.

◆ Use the mouse techniques of pointing, clicking, double-clicking, and dragging.

◆ Identify the parts of a window.

◆ Move, size, and alter the view of a window.

◆ Identify the parts of a dialog box.

◆ Perform common tasks, such as starting a program, selecting a menu command, using shortcut menus, accessing online help, and shutting down Windows 95.

KEY TERMS

applications software
check box
clicking
command button
counter button
defaults
dialog box
double-clicking
dragging
drop-down list box
folders
icons
menu bar

pointer
pointing
radio button
scroll bar
shortcut icons
shortcut menus
system software
tabs
taskbar
text box
title bar
triangle button
window

INTRODUCTION TO WINDOWS 95

Computer systems consist of hardware and software. Hardware includes the physical parts of the computer system—those that are visible, including the monitor, keyboard, processor, printer, and mouse. Software consists of sets of instructions or programs that tell the hardware what to do. The two most important types of software are system software and applications software.

system software *a program that controls critical functions of a computer.*

System software, also known as the operating system, performs a number of critical functions: it controls the flow of information between different hardware components, enables programs to run smoothly, and determines the look and feel of the information on screen to the user. Windows 95 is one example of system software. Not all computers use the same operating system; before Windows was released, many computers used the Disk Operating System (DOS).

applications software *a program designed to perform specific tasks.*

Applications software is designed to perform specific tasks. For example, Microsoft Word is a popular applications software program used for word processing. MediSoft for Windows is another example of an applications program. It is designed to perform billing and scheduling in a medical office.

Windows 95 uses what is called a graphical user interface (GUI). A graphical user interface is a type of computer operating system in which commands are carried out by responding to visual information on the screen. While the term may be cumbersome, the program is not. In fact, most users find Windows 95 relatively easy to use.

WINDOWS 95 TECHNIQUES

Pointer

In Windows 95, a device known as a mouse is used to interact with information displayed on the screen. By pointing to items on the screen and clicking one of the mouse buttons, commands are issued without using the keyboard. There are a few basic techniques that are essential to working successfully with Windows 95. These include pointing, clicking, double-clicking, and dragging.

POINTING

pointer *an arrow displayed on the screen that moves when the mouse is moved.*

The **pointer** is an arrow that appears on the screen. This pointer represents the mouse. When the mouse moves, the pointer on the screen moves with it. If the mouse is moved to the left, the pointer moves to the left. If the mouse is moved away from the user, the

CLICKING

pointing the corresponding movement between the mouse and the pointer.

pointer moves up toward the top of the screen. This movement of the mouse and the corresponding movement of the pointer on the screen is called **pointing**.

Pointing is associated with clicking. **Clicking** refers to the activity of pressing and releasing a button on the mouse, usually the left mouse button. The result of clicking varies depending on the activity being performed. Most of the time clicking is used to activate a command. For example, if the pointer is positioned on the File menu, clicking opens the menu. If the pointer is then positioned on the Save command that is located on the File menu, clicking executes the command.

Pointing and clicking can be used to highlight an icon or text. When an item is highlighted, it changes color. It may become darker, such as when an icon is selected. Or, in the case of highlighting text, it may appear as white type on a colored bar. (For example, see Figure 3-4 on page 35. The Select All command is highlighted.) Highlighting indicates that the chosen item is the object of the next action. For example, if an icon on the desktop is highlighted, it can be opened, copied, moved, and so on. If a line of text in a word processing document is highlighted, it can be cut, copied, and so on. A highlighted item is the currently active item. Only one item can be active at a time; an item remains active until another item is highlighted or until another item or area of the desktop is clicked.

DOUBLE-CLICKING

double-clicking clicking the left mouse button twice in rapid succession.

While some Windows commands are executed by pointing and clicking, others require double-clicking. This latter technique is used frequently to open windows and programs. **Double-clicking** is a technique in which the left mouse button is clicked twice in rapid succession while the pointer points to an object. Double-clicking is not the same as clicking the mouse button twice. In double-clicking, the button must be clicked very rapidly. If the clicks are too slow (too far apart in time), the command will not be executed.

DRAGGING

dragging moving an object around the desktop by holding down the left mouse button and moving the mouse.

Objects can be moved around the desktop using a technique called **dragging**. To drag an object, point to it with the pointer, hold down the left mouse button, and move the mouse until the object appears in the new location.

STARTING AND SHUTTING DOWN WINDOWS 95

STARTING WINDOWS 95

The following steps are used to start Windows 95:

1. Turn on the computer. If the monitor has a separate on/off, switch, turn the monitor on.

2. Wait while the computer goes through the process of starting up, known as booting.

3. When the booting process is finished, the Windows 95 desktop appears. On some computers, a Welcome window is also displayed on the Windows 95 desktop.

SHUTTING DOWN WINDOWS 95

A series of steps must be followed when it is time to shut down the computer. If any applications are in use, the data within them should be saved before the applications are exited. Then, the Start button is clicked (bottom-left corner of the Windows 95 desktop), and the Shut Down command is selected. The Shut Down Windows dialog box is displayed, as shown in Figure 3-1. This dialog box asks whether the user wants to:

◆ Shut down the computer

◆ Restart the computer

◆ Restart the computer in MS-DOS mode

To shut down the computer, the button next to the option labeled "Shut down the computer?" is clicked. Then the Yes button is clicked. Windows 95 displays a message asking the user to wait while the system shuts down. A second message appears when it is safe to turn off the power to the computer.

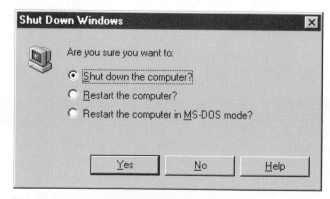

Figure 3-1 Shut Down Windows dialog box.

THE WINDOWS 95 DESKTOP

The Windows 95 desktop is similar to a desktop in an office. There are a number of items on the desktop. The items on the desktop vary depending on how the computer is set up and what programs are installed. However, several items are common to all Windows 95 desktops—these include icons and the taskbar (see Figure 3-2).

ICONS

icons visual symbols that represent files, folders, devices, and programs.

window a box that displays information on screen.

Icons are visual symbols that represent files, folders, devices, and programs. The contents of an icon can be viewed by double-clicking the icon. This opens a window that displays the icon's contents. A **window** is a box that displays information on screen. Icons common to most Windows 95 desktops include the My Computer and Recycle Bin icons.

My Computer   Clicking the My Computer icon displays a window listing the contents of the computer, including the hard drive, the CD-ROM drive, and the floppy drive.

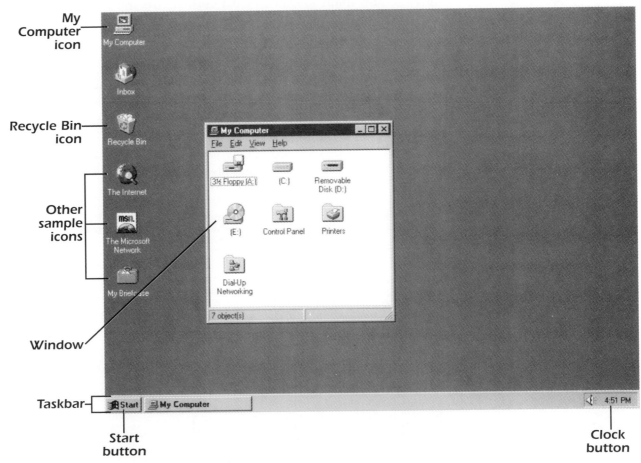

Figure 3-2 A sample Windows 95 desktop.

Recycle Bin Clicking the Recycle Bin icon displays a window from which files, programs, and icons that are no longer needed can be deleted. When files are deleted in Windows 95, they are stored in the Recycle Bin until the Recycle Bin is emptied.

shortcut icons *visual symbols that represent commonly used programs.*

Icons for application programs may also appear on the Windows 95 desktop. These application icons are known as **shortcut icons**. Double-clicking a shortcut icon launches an application program directly from the desktop.

TASKBAR

taskbar *a bar located at the bottom of the desktop. It contains several buttons, including the Start button and the Clock button.*

The **taskbar** is located at the bottom of the desktop. The Start button and the Clock button are located on the taskbar. The Start button is used to locate and launch applications. The Clock button displays the current time. It is used to set the system date and time. Any other currently running application programs are displayed as buttons on the taskbar.

WINDOWS

All of the work performed in Windows 95 is completed in windows. Windows can be opened, closed, minimized, maximized, sized, and moved. The main features of a window are the title bar and the menu bar (see Figure 3-3).

Title Bar

title bar *the band at the top of a window that lists the name of the window.*

The **title bar** is the band at the top of the window that lists the name of the window. When the title bar appears in a color, such as blue, it indicates that this window is the active window. An active window

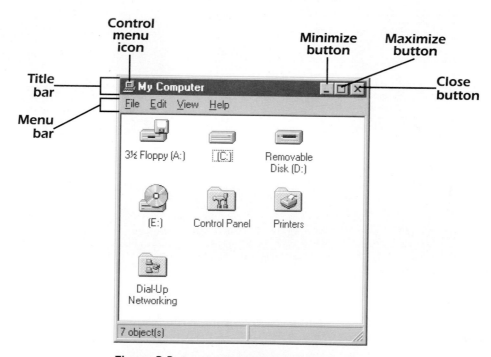

Figure 3-3 A sample My Computer window.

is one that is ready for input, either from the keyboard or the mouse. More than one window may be open on the desktop at one time. Windows can overlap each other. However, only one window can be active at one time. A window that is open but not the active window is called an inactive window. A window is made active by clicking on it once with the left mouse button.

The title bar also contains an icon and a series of buttons. These are listed in Table 3-1.

Table 3-1   Title Bar Icon and Buttons

Icon/Button	Name	Activity
![Control menu icon]	Control menu icon	Contains options for moving, sizing, and closing the window.
![Minimize button]	Minimize button	Reduces the window to a button on the taskbar.
![Maximize button]	Maximize button	Expands the window to fill the entire screen.
![Close button]	Close button	Closes the window.

Menu Bar

menu bar a bar located beneath the title bar. It lists the names of the menus available in the window.

Located just beneath the title bar, the **menu bar** lists the names of the menus available in the window. To display the contents of a menu, point to the menu name and click the left mouse button. The options listed on a menu are known as menu commands (see Figure 3-4). Not all menu commands are available all the time. All commands

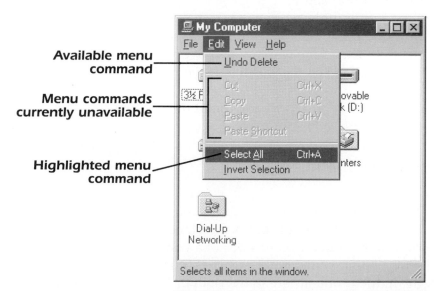

Figure 3-4 Sample window with drop-down menu displayed.

are listed, but some may be dimmed. A dimmed menu command is currently unavailable. Commands are usually dimmed when they are not appropriate to the task being performed. For example, if the Edit menu is accessed but no file was previously selected for editing, many commands on the menu will appear dimmed. When a file is selected for editing, those menu commands will appear in dark letters and may be selected.

WORKING WITH WINDOWS

Information is displayed on the computer's screen in a window. To use Windows 95 effectively, it is important to know how to work with these windows, including how to move a window, resize a window, and change what is displayed in a window.

MOVING A WINDOW

Windows can be moved anywhere on the desktop. To move a window, point to the title bar and drag the window to the desired location while holding down the left mouse button. While dragging the window, only its outline moves. When the mouse button is released, the window appears in its new location.

SIZING A WINDOW

The size and shape of a window can be changed. When the pointer is placed on the edge of a window, its appearance changes from a pointer to a type of pointer with double-headed arrows. When the pointer is placed at the right or left edge of the window, it becomes a horizontal double-headed arrow. When the pointer is placed at the top or bottom edge of the window, it becomes a vertical double-headed arrow.

Resizing pointers

When the pointer is a double-headed arrow, holding down the left mouse button and dragging the mouse changes the size of the window. For example, positioning the pointer on the left edge of the window and dragging to the left makes the window wider; dragging to the right makes the window narrower. Similarly, the window can be lengthened or shortened using the vertical double-headed arrow.

To size the vertical and horizontal dimensions simultaneously, the pointer is placed in one of the four corners of the window. Dragging inward reduces the size of the window; dragging outward increases the window size.

CHANGING WHAT IS DISPLAYED IN A WINDOW

scroll bar a rectangular bar that appears on the right or bottom (or both) sides of a window.

To change the information displayed within a window, the scroll bars are used. A **scroll bar** is a rectangular bar that appears on the right or bottom (or both) sides of a window that is too small to display all of its contents at one time. If the window is too narrow and the hidden contents are to the right or left of what is visible, a scroll bar appears on the bottom of the window. If the window is too short and the hidden contents are above or below what is visible, a scroll bar appears at the right of the window.

Scroll bars contain scroll boxes and scroll arrows (see Figure 3-5). All three tools—the scroll bars, the scroll boxes, and the scroll arrows—can be used to change the view in a window.

Using the Scroll Bar   To change the view using the scroll bar, click in an area of the bar. The view changes to display information that was not previously visible.

Using the Scroll Box   To change the view using the scroll box, the scroll box is dragged to another position. For example, if the scroll box is positioned at the top of the scroll bar, the window displays the

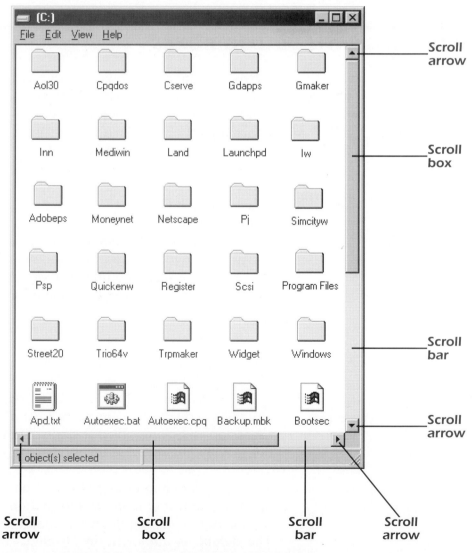

Figure 3-5 *Sample window showing scrolling tools.*

contents located in the top section of the window. If the scroll box is dragged to the center of the scroll bar, the window displays the contents in the center of the window. The same is true for the scroll box located at the bottom of the window. When a scroll box is positioned all the way to the left, the contents on the left side of the window are displayed. When it is dragged all the way to the right, the contents on the right are displayed.

Using the Scroll Arrows The view of the window can also be changed using the scroll arrows on each scroll bar. There are two arrows on each scroll bar, one at either end. When a scroll arrow is clicked, the scroll box moves a small increment in the direction the arrow points. For example, if the left scroll arrow is clicked, the scroll box shifts an increment to the left, as do the contents displayed in the window.

WORKING WITH DIALOG BOXES

dialog box a window that appears on screen requesting more information from the user.

When certain commands are selected, a window appears that requests more information from the person using the computer. This window is called a **dialog box** because it asks for an exchange of information between two parties: the computer and the user. For example, a dialog box for the Print command might ask how many copies of a document are to be printed.

Other dialog boxes are requests for confirmation. For example, if a command was given to delete a file, a dialog box would ask for confirmation that the file should be deleted. Dialog boxes are used to perform many activities in Windows 95 application programs. Dialog boxes contain a number of options for entering information (see Figure 3-6). The most common options are listed below.

TEXT BOX

text box a box in which information is entered.

defaults standard values used by the software.

A **text box** is a box in which information is entered. For the purpose of this text/workbook, because the term is used so often, "text box" is generally shortened to "box." The box may be blank, or it may already have letters or numbers in it. If the box already contains characters, these are called defaults. **Defaults** are the standard values used by the software unless the user enters different values.

To enter information in a blank text box, click in the box and then key the characters. To enter information in a text box that contains the default value, highlight the characters and key the new entry. The default is automatically deleted. Another way of deleting a default value is to highlight the entry and press the Delete key.

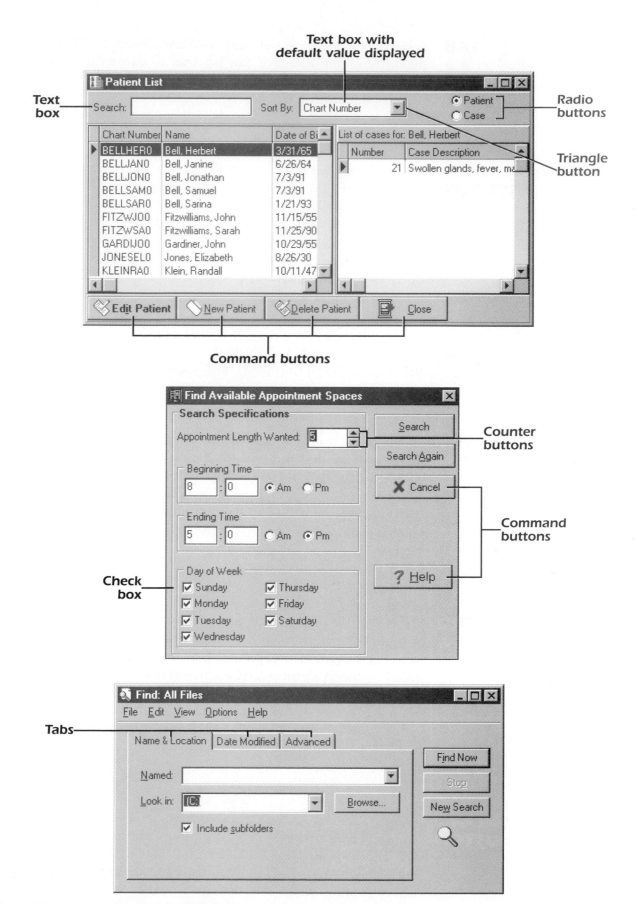

Figure 3-6 Sample dialog boxes (MediSoft).

TAB

tabs subsets of options within a dialog box.

Some dialog boxes contain **tabs**. Tabs are subsets of options within a dialog box. The name of the tab that is currently active usually appears in boldfaced type. To make a different tab active, click the name of the desired tab.

DROP-DOWN LIST BOX

drop-down list box a box that contains a predetermined list of options.

triangle button a button used to display the contents of a drop-down list.

A **drop-down list box** is a box that contains a predetermined list of options. The first entry in the list is displayed. To see the other options, a small triangle button to the right of the box must be clicked. The **triangle button** is used to display the contents of the drop-down list. When the button is clicked, the list "drops-down" and all the options become visible. To select an item from the drop-down list, simply click on it.

CHECK BOX

check box a box used to turn options on and off.

A **check box** is used to turn an option on and off. If the option is off, the box is blank. If the option is on, a check mark (✓) or "X" appears.

COUNTER BUTTON

counter button a button used to change a numerical entry.

A **counter button** is used to change a numerical entry, such as a year. Two small counter buttons are shown to the right of a text box in Figure 3-6 (page 39). The counter button on the top displays a small triangle pointing up, and the button on the bottom contains a triangle pointing down. To increase the numerical value in the text box, the top button is clicked. To decrease the value, the bottom button is clicked.

RADIO BUTTON

radio button a button used to select between a number of options.

A **radio button** is a small round button that is used to select between a number of options. For example, radio buttons can be used to select between a.m. and p.m., or between male and female. Only one radio button in a group can be active at one time. Selecting one radio button automatically deselects the other button(s). When a radio button is active, it has a solid black dot in the middle. If it is not active, the center is blank. To select a radio button, click on the button of the desired option.

COMMAND BUTTON

command button a button used to activate commands.

After options are selected and/or data is keyed in a dialog box, a **command button** is clicked. Common command buttons include OK and Cancel. The OK button indicates that it is all right to go ahead with the selections made in the dialog box. Clicking the Cancel button closes the dialog box without making any of the changes just entered.

PERFORMING COMMON TASKS IN WINDOWS 95

This section describes how to perform four of the most common tasks in Windows 95: starting a program, selecting a menu command, using shortcut menus, and accessing online help.

STARTING A PROGRAM

folders *locations on screen in which files are stored.*

Windows organizes the files on the computer into folders. **Folders** are used to store different types of files. The Programs folder contains the software programs that are installed on the computer. The Programs folder is accessed through the Start button, located on the taskbar. When the Start button is clicked, the Start menu appears. The Start menu lists a number of folders and icons, including the Programs folder. When the pointer is placed on the Programs folder, a submenu is displayed. This submenu lists folders for the programs installed on this computer. For example, if the MediSoft program is installed, a MediSoft program folder appears on the submenu (see Figure 3-7). When the pointer is placed on the program folder, another submenu appears. This submenu displays the icon(s) for the program. Clicking on a program icon starts the program.

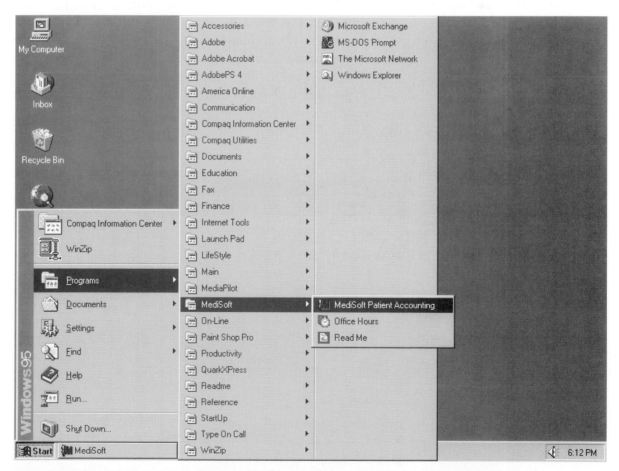

Figure 3-7 *Sample Start menu showing the Programs and MediSoft folders selected.*

SELECTING A MENU COMMAND

One of the most common tasks performed in Windows is selecting a menu command. There are several ways of selecting a menu command. Using the mouse, point to the menu name and click the left mouse button. The menu appears, listing all the possible commands. When the mouse is moved and is pointing to a menu command, that command is highlighted. The menu command name is displayed in white instead of a color, and a colored band extends through the name. To select a menu command, click on the command while it is highlighted using the left mouse button.

There are also ways of selecting menu commands using the keyboard. Each menu command contains one underlined letter. To select this command using the keyboard, the Alt key is held down while the underlined key is pressed. For example, to select the File menu, Alt + F would be pressed.

Menu commands can also be selected using the up and down arrow keys to highlight the desired command. Once the command is highlighted, there are two ways of activating it. One way is to press the Enter key; the other way is to press the key of the underlined letter.

USING SHORTCUT MENUS

shortcut menus *menus containing commonly used commands.*

Shortcut menus are lists of the most commonly used commands (see Figure 3-8). For example, a shortcut menu in MediSoft offers commands for editing, deleting, or creating a new patient record. Shortcut menus are accessed by pointing to an object and clicking the *right* mouse button. To execute a command on the menu, point and click. To close a shortcut menu without choosing any command, click on something in the window other than the menu.

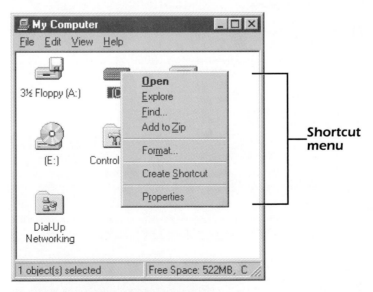

Figure 3-8 *Sample shortcut menu.*

ACCESSING ONLINE HELP

Windows 95 provides an online help feature, which is accessed by clicking the Start button and clicking Help on the Start menu. When the Help command is selected, the Help Topics dialog box appears. The first tab in the dialog box is labeled "Contents" (see Figure 3-9). The Contents tab lists several help topics available, such as "How To…" and "Troubleshooting." It also lists other options including a tour of Windows 95 for new users, and a list of commonly asked questions and their answers for those users who have previously worked with Windows. To select a topic listed on the Contents tab, click the topic and then click the bottom-left command button. Depending on the topic chosen, the button will read "Display" or "Open."

The second tab in the Help Topics dialog box is the Index tab (see Figure 3-10 on page 44). This tab provides a comprehensive listing of all help topics available in online help. It also provides a search option. To locate help on a particular topic, scroll down the list of topics, or enter a word or phrase in the blank text box at the top of the dialog box. As soon as a letter is entered, the computer scrolls down the list to the topic that most closely matches what has been keyed in the search box. For example, if "w" is entered in the search box, the first entry in the list that begins with the letter "w" is highlighted. When the desired topic is highlighted, clicking the Display

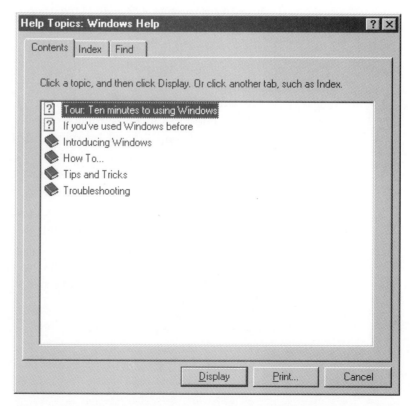

Figure 3-9 Help Topics dialog box with Contents tab displayed.

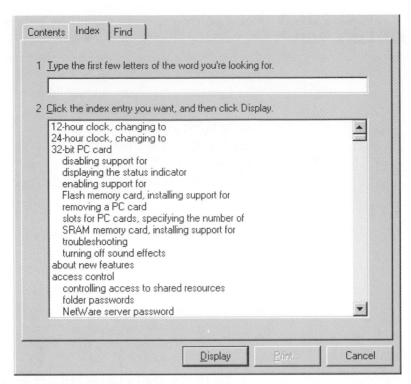

Figure 3-10 Index tab.

button opens the Windows Help dialog box. (If the topic is complex, clicking the Display button may first display another dialog box, with a subset of topics. If this happens, click the topic of interest from the subset and then click the Display button.)

The third tab in the Help Topics dialog box is the Find tab (see Figure 3-11a). The Find tab is similar to the Index tab, except in the Find tab topics are organized not by name but by topic. For example, to discover how to copy the contents of a window using the Index tab, it would be necessary to look under the topic of "window," and then under the subentry "copying window contents." In the Find tab, help would be found under the topic "Copying the window or screen contents." To access help in the Find tab, search for a topic by entering text in the search box, or select a topic by scrolling through the list. When the topic of interest is highlighted, click the Display button to view the help information in the Windows Help dialog box (see Figure 3-11b).

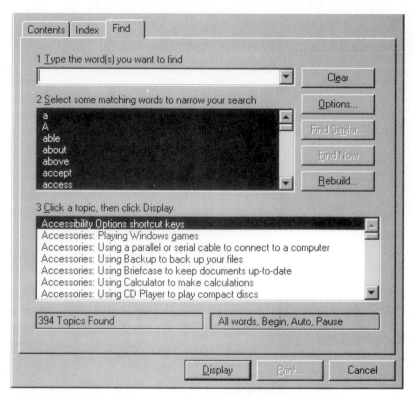

Figure 3-11a Find tab.

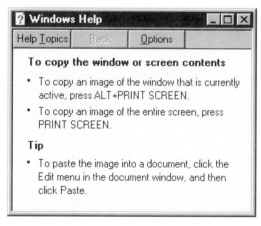

Figure 3-11b Windows Help dialog box.

CHAPTER REVIEW

USING TERMINOLOGY

Match the terms on the left with the definitions on the right.

_____ 1. applications software

_____ 2. check box

_____ 3. clicking

_____ 4. command button

_____ 5. counter button

_____ 6. defaults

_____ 7. dialog box

_____ 8. double-clicking

_____ 9. dragging

_____ 10. drop-down list box

_____ 11. folders

_____ 12. icons

_____ 13. menu bar

_____ 14. pointer

_____ 15. pointing

_____ 16. radio button

a. A program that controls critical functions of a computer.

b. Subsets of options within a dialog box.

c. Programs designed to perform specific tasks.

d. A box that contains a predetermined list of options.

e. A button used to display the contents of a drop-down list.

f. Visual symbols that represent files, folders, devices, and programs.

g. A box that displays information on screen.

h. The band at the top of a window that lists the name of the window.

i. A box used to turn options on and off.

j. An arrow displayed on the screen that moves when the mouse is moved.

k. A button used to change a numerical entry.

l. Visual symbols that represent commonly used programs.

m. A bar located at the bottom of the desktop. It contains several buttons, including the Start button and the Clock button.

n. Standard values used by the software.

o. A button used to select between a number of options.

p. A bar located beneath the title bar. It lists the names of the menus available in the window.

_____ **17.** scroll bar

_____ **18.** shortcut icons

_____ **19.** shortcut menus

_____ **20.** system software

_____ **21.** tabs

_____ **22.** taskbar

_____ **23.** text box

_____ **24.** title bar

_____ **25.** triangle button

_____ **26.** window

q. The corresponding movement between the mouse and the pointer.

r. Clicking the left mouse button twice in rapid succession.

s. Menus containing commonly used commands.

t. A rectangular bar that appears on the right or bottom (or both) sides of a window.

u. A window that appears on screen requesting more information from the user.

v. Moving an object around the desktop by holding down the left mouse button and moving the mouse.

w. A button used to activate commands.

x. A box in which information is entered.

y. Pressing and releasing a button on the mouse.

z. Locations on screen in which files are stored.

CHECKING YOUR UNDERSTANDING

27. Label the parts of a window on the lines provided.

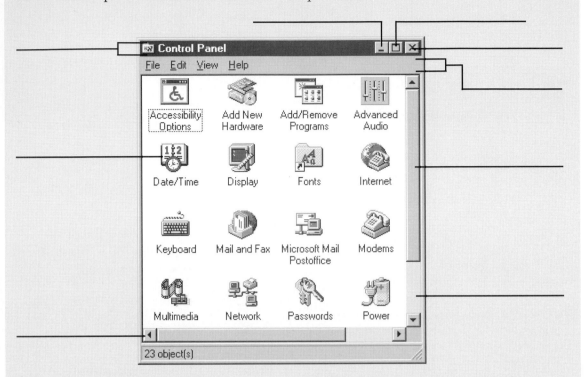

28. Label the parts of a dialog box on the lines provided.

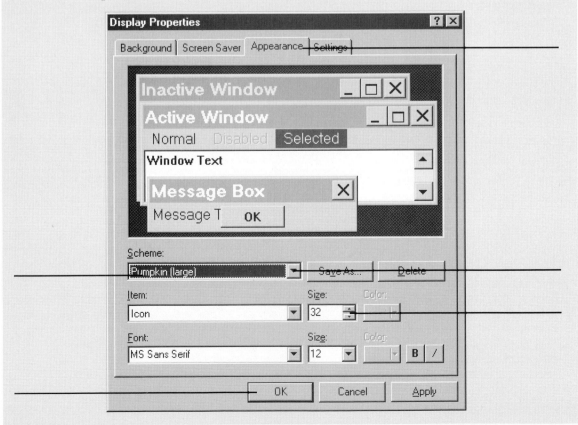

AT THE COMPUTER

Complete the following activities at the computer:

29. Start Windows 95 and practice using the scroll bars and menus:

  a. Start Windows 95.

  b. Open the My Computer window.

  c. If scroll bars are not visible on the right side and the bottom of the window, resize the window to make it approximately 2" high x 3" wide.

  d. Practice using the scroll bars to see contents of the window that are not visible.

  e. Open the Edit menu.

  f. Point to the Select All command, and click the left mouse button. Notice that all the icons in the My Computer window are highlighted.

  g. Close the My Computer window.

30. Click Help on the Start menu to access the Windows 95 online Help feature. Search for help on the topic of making a copy of a floppy disk by completing the following steps:

  a. Click the Find tab to make it active.

  b. Key *disks* in the "1 Type the word(s) you want to find" box.

  c. Click "Making a copy of a floppy disk" in the "3 Click a topic, then click Display" box.

  d. Click the Display button. The Windows Help dialog box is displayed.

  e. Read the contents of the Windows Help dialog box.

  f. Close the Windows Help dialog box.

MediSoft for Windows Training

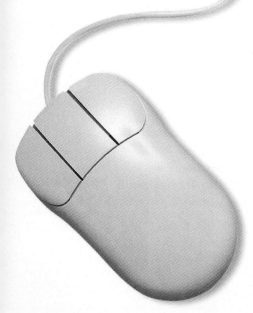

CHAPTER 4
Introduction to MediSoft

WHAT YOU NEED TO KNOW

To use this chapter, you need to know how to:
- ◆ Start your computer and Microsoft for Windows.
- ◆ Use the keyboard and mouse.

OBJECTIVES

In this chapter, you will learn how to:
- ◆ Start MediSoft.
- ◆ Use the Student Data Disk.
- ◆ Move around the MediSoft menus.
- ◆ Use the MediSoft toolbar.
- ◆ Enter, edit, and delete data in MediSoft.
- ◆ Save and back up MediSoft data.
- ◆ Use MediSoft's Online Help features.
- ◆ Exit MediSoft.

KEY TERMS

backup data
balloon help
MMDDCCYY format

MMDDYY format
transactions

WHAT IS MEDISOFT?

MediSoft is a patient accounting software program. Information on patients, providers, insurance carriers, and patient and insurance billing is stored and processed by the system. MediSoft is widely used by medical practices throughout the United States. It is typically used to accomplish the following daily work in a medical practice:

◆ Enter information on new patients, and change information on established patients as needed.
◆ Enter transactions, such as charges, to patients' accounts.
◆ Record payments and adjustments from patients and insurance companies.
◆ Print walkout receipts and statements for patients.
◆ Submit insurance claims to carriers.
◆ Print standard reports, and create custom reports.
◆ Schedule appointments.

Many of the general working concepts used in operating MediSoft are similar to those in other software programs. Thus, you should be able to transfer many skills taught in this text/workbook about MediSoft to other patient accounting programs.

HOW MEDISOFT DATA IS ORGANIZED AND STORED

Information entered into MediSoft is stored in databases. As defined in Chapter 2, a database is a collection of related pieces of information.

MEDISOFT DATABASES

MediSoft stores these major types of data:

◆ **Provider Data** The provider database has information about the physician(s) as well as the practice, such as its name and address, phone number, and tax and medical identifier numbers.
◆ **Patient Data** Each patient information form is stored in the computer system's patient database. The patient's unique chart number and personal information—name and address, phone number, birth date, Social Security number, gender, marital status, and employer—are examples of information stored in this database.
◆ **Insurance Carriers** The insurance carrier database contains the names, addresses, and other data about each insurance carrier used by patients, such as the type of plan. Usually, this database also records information on each carrier's electronic media claim (EMC) submission.
◆ **Diagnosis Codes** The diagnosis code database contains the *International Classification of Diseases, 9th Revision, Clinical Modification (ICD-9)* codes that indicate the reason a service is provided. The codes entered in this database are those most frequently used by the practice. The practice's superbill often serves as a source document when the MediSoft system is first set up.

- **Procedure Codes** The procedure code database contains the data needed to create charges. The *Physicians' Current Procedural Terminology (CPT)* codes most often used by the practice are selected for this database. The practice's superbill is often a good source document for these codes. Other claim data elements, such as place of service (POS) and the charge for each procedure, are stored in the procedure code database.
- **Transactions** The transaction database stores information about each patient's visits, diagnoses, and procedures, as well as received and outstanding payments. **Transactions** in the form of charges, payments, and adjustments are also stored in the transaction database.

transactions charges, payments, and adjustments.

Within MediSoft, each database is linked, or related, to each of the others by having at least one fact in common. For example, information entered in the patient database is shared with the transaction database, linking the two. Information is entered only once; MediSoft selects the data from each database as needed.

USING THE STUDENT DATA DISK

Before a medical office begins using MediSoft, basic information about the practice and its patients must be entered in the computer. For the exercises you will complete in this text/workbook, this preliminary work has been done for you. The MediSoft databases are stored on the Student Data Disk located inside the back cover.

The Student Data Disk contains a folder that includes the data for the practice used in this text/workbook, the Family Care Center (FCC). Before you begin using the Student Data Disk, you need to make a working copy of it using the instructions below. When you are finished making the disk copy, store the original Student Data Disk in a safe place. You may need to use this disk to make another copy if the working disk is accidentally damaged or lost.

Complete the following steps to make a copy of the Student Data Disk. If your computer has a version of Windows other than Windows 95, ask your instructor for alternate directions.

1. Turn on the computer and monitor.

2. After the Windows 95 desktop is displayed, insert the Student Data Disk in the 3½ floppy drive (Drive A).

3. Double-click the My Computer icon on the desktop. The My Computer window is displayed.

4. Click the icon labeled "3½ Floppy (A:)."

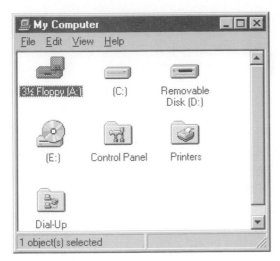

Sample My Computer window with
3½ Floppy (A:) icon highlighted.

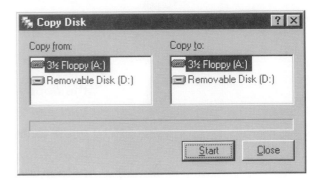

Copy Disk dialog box.

5. On the File menu, click Copy Disk. The Copy Disk dialog box is displayed.

6. The Copy From and Copy To windows should have "3½ Floppy (A:)" highlighted. If they are not highlighted, click 3½ Floppy (A:) in both the Copy From and Copy To windows.

7. Click the Start button. The computer begins reading the files on the source disk. You can monitor the computer's progress by viewing the bar above the words "Reading source disk."

8. When the system prompts you to insert the disk you want to copy to (the destination disk), eject the Student Data Disk from the drive.

9. Insert a blank disk in the floppy drive, and click the OK button. The files are copied to the destination disk. Again, you can monitor the progress by looking at the bar above the words "Writing to destination disk."

10. When the copy is completed, the message "Copy completed successfully" is displayed. Eject the disk from the drive and label it "Working Copy FCC."

11. Close the My Computer dialog box by clicking the Close button.

USING MEDISOFT

To begin using MediSoft, it is necessary to have a basic understanding of how to start the program; enter, edit, and save data; and exit the program. This section provides that information.

The following exercise describes how to start the MediSoft program.

Exercise 4-1

To start MediSoft, follow these steps. (Steps 6 through 12 may only occur the first time you enter MediSoft after installation.)

1. Turn on the computer and monitor.

2. Insert the Student Data Disk labeled "Working Copy FCC" in the floppy drive.

3. Click the Start button on the Windows 95 taskbar.

4. Point to Programs. A pop-up menu is displayed to the right.

5. Point to MediSoft. Click MediSoft Patient Accounting on the pop-up menu.

6. MediSoft opens and displays the Create Data dialog box. Click the top button to create a new set of data. The Create a New Set of Data dialog box is displayed.

7. Key *Family Care Center* in the box labeled "Enter the practice or doctors name to identify this set of data."

8. Press the Tab key. The information in the box labeled "Enter the data path" is highlighted. Click the Delete key to eliminate the default data path.

9. Key *A:\FCC* in the data path box.

10. Click the Create button. Do not be alarmed by the warning message that is displayed next; it is normal.

11. Click the Yes button. The Practice Information dialog box is displayed.

12. Click the Save button. Your screen should look like the one shown in Figure 4-1. If a name other than Family Care Center displays on the title bar at the top of the screen, ask your instructor for assistance.

THE MEDISOFT MENU BAR

MediSoft offers choices of actions through a series of menus. Commands are issued by clicking an option on the menu bar or by clicking a shortcut button on the toolbar. The menu bar lists the names of the menus in MediSoft: File, Edit, Activities, Lists, Reports, Tools, Window, and Help (see Figure 4-2). Beneath each menu name is a pull-down menu of one or more options.

File Menu   The File menu is used to enter information about the medical office practice when first setting up MediSoft. It is also used to back up data, maintain files, and set program options (see Figure 4-3).

Edit Menu   The Edit menu contains the basic commands needed to move, change, or delete information (see Figure 4-4). These commands are Undo, Cut, Copy, Paste, and Delete.

Activities Menu   Most medical office data collected on a day-to-day basis is entered through options on the Activities menu (see Figure 4-5). This menu is used to enter information about patients'

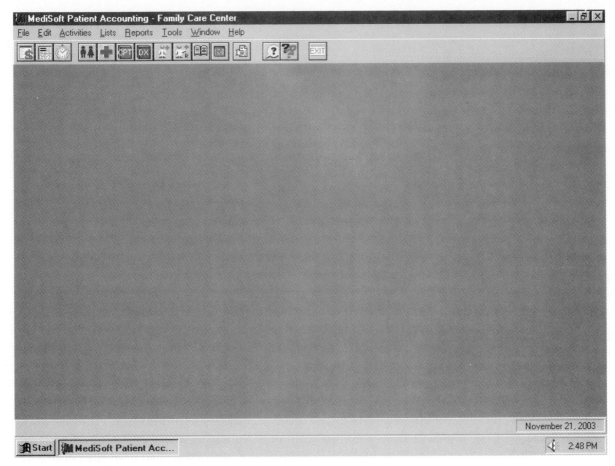

Figure 4-1 MediSoft opening screen.

File   Edit   Activities   Lists   Reports   Tools   Window   Help

Figure 4-2 MediSoft menu bar.

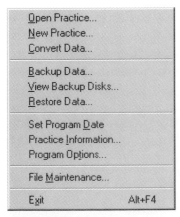

Figure 4-3 File menu.

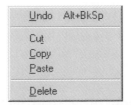

Figure 4-4 Edit menu.

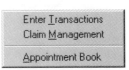

Figure 4-5 Activities menu.

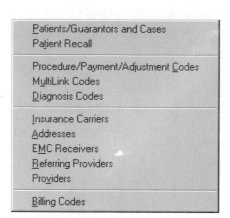

Figure 4-6 Lists menu.

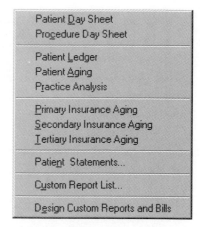

Figure 4-7 Reports menu.

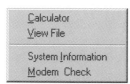

Figure 4-8 Tools menu.

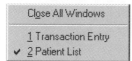

Figure 4-9 Window menu.

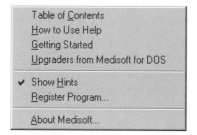

Figure 4-10 Help menu.

office visits, including diagnoses, and procedures performed. Transactions, including charges, payments, and adjustments, are also entered via the Activities menu. The Activities menu also includes the Claim Management option for processing insurance claims. Office Hours, MediSoft's built-in appointment scheduler, is another option on this menu, labeled "Appointment Book."

Lists Menu Information on new patients, such as name, address, and employer, is entered through the Lists menu (see Figure 4-6). If information needs to be changed on an established patient, it is also updated through this menu. The Lists menu also provides access to lists of codes, insurance carriers, and providers. These lists may be updated and printed when necessary.

Reports Menu The Reports menu is used to print reports about patients' accounts and other reports about the practice (see Figure 4-7).

Tools Menu The calculator is accessed through the Tools menu. Other options on the Tools menu can be used to view the contents of a file as well as a profile of the computer system (see Figure 4-8).

Window Menu Using the Window menu, it is possible to switch back and forth between several open windows. For example, if the Transaction Entry dialog box and the Patient List dialog box were both open, the Window menu would look like the menu in Figure 4-9. The Window menu also has an option to close all windows.

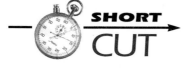

The easiest way to switch back and forth between two or more open windows is to click anywhere on a window to make it the active window. Clicking on a window makes it active and automatically deselects the other previously active window.

Help Menu The Help menu, shown in Figure 4-10, is used to access MediSoft's Help feature.

Exercise 4-2

Practice using the menus.

1. Click the Lists menu on the menu bar.

2. Click Patients/Guarantors and Cases. The Patient List dialog box is displayed (see Figure 4-11).

3. Click the Close button at the bottom of the dialog box.

4. Click the Activities menu.

5. Click Enter Transactions. The Transaction Entry dialog box is displayed (see Figure 4-12).

6. Click the Close button.

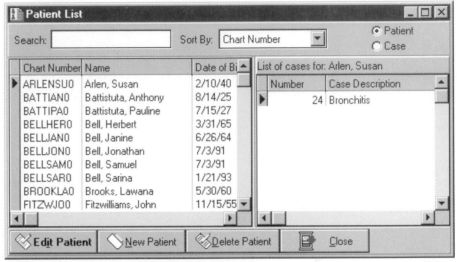

Figure 4-11 Patient List dialog box.

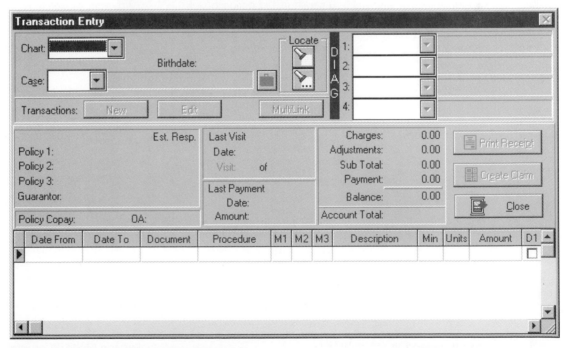

Figure 4-12 Transaction Entry dialog box.

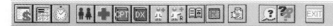

Figure 4-13 MediSoft toolbar.

THE MEDISOFT TOOLBAR

Located below the menu bar, the toolbar contains a series of buttons with icons that represent the most common activities performed in MediSoft. These buttons are shortcuts for frequently used menu commands. The toolbar displays 15 buttons (see Figure 4-13).

Table 4-1   Toolbar Buttons

Button	Button Name	Associated Function	Activity
	Transaction Entry	Transaction Entry dialog box	Enter transactions.
	Claim Management	Claim Management dialog box	Create and send insurance claims.
	Appointment Book	Office Hours	Schedule appointments.
	Patient List	Patient List dialog box	Enter and edit patient information.
	Insurance Carrier List	Insurance Carrier List dialog box	Add, edit, or delete insurance carriers.
	Procedure Code List	Procedure/Payment/Adjustment List dialog box	Add, edit, or delete procedure, payment, and adjustment codes.
	Diagnosis Code List	Diagnosis List dialog box	Add, edit, or delete diagnosis codes.
	Provider List	Provider List dialog box	Add, edit, or delete providers.
	Referring Provider List	Referring Provider List dialog box	Add, edit, or delete referring providers.
	Address List	Address List dialog box	Add, edit, or delete addresses.
	Patient Recall Entry	Patient Recall dialog box	Add a patient to the recall list.
	Custom Report List	Open Report dialog box	Display or print reports.
	Show/Hide Hints	Balloon help	Turn the Hints feature on or off.
	Help	Contents dialog box	Access MediSoft's online help files.
	Exit the MediSoft Program	Exit	Exit the MediSoft program.

Exercise 4-3

Practice using buttons on the toolbar.

1. Click the Provider List button. The Provider List dialog box is displayed (see Figure 4-14).

2. Click the Close button to close the dialog box.

3. Click the Procedure Code List button. The Procedure/ Payment/ Adjustment List dialog box is displayed (see Figure 4-15).

4. Click the Close button to close the dialog box.

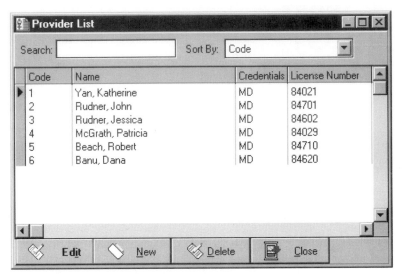

Figure 4-14 Provider List dialog box.

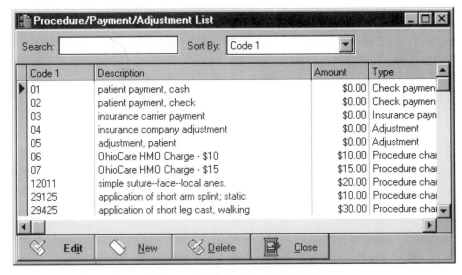

Figure 4-15 Procedure/Payment/Adjustment dialog box.

ENTERING AND EDITING DATA

All data, whether a patient's address or a charge for a procedure, are entered into MediSoft through the menus on the menu bar or through the buttons on the toolbar. Selecting an option from the menus or toolbar brings up a dialog box. The Tab key is used to move between text boxes within a dialog box. In some dialog boxes, information is entered by keying data into a text box. For example, a patient's name would be keyed directly into a text box. At other times selections are made from a list of choices already present. For example, when entering the name of the provider a patient is seeing, the provider is selected from a drop-down list of providers already in the system.

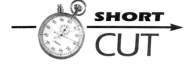

To make a selection from a drop-down list, either of these techniques can be used: the scroll bars can be used to scroll up or down the list until the desired entry is displayed, or, the first few letters of the desired entry can be keyed in the text box next to the drop-down list. When characters are keyed, the system displays the entry in the list that most closely matches the characters keyed. When the desired entry appears highlighted, the Enter key is pressed. In most instances, the latter method is much quicker than using the scroll bars to locate the desired entry. Imagine a practice with 3000 patients. To locate a patient named Zawacki using the scroll method would require scrolling down a very long list. Keying in the first few letters of the patient's chart number, in this case "ZAW," would cause the system to display the first entry beginning with those letters. (Chart numbers are discussed in Chapter 5.)

Dates

MediSoft is a date-sensitive program that uses two dates: the MediSoft Program Date and the Windows System Date. The dates set in MediSoft and Windows must be accurate, or the data entered will be of little value to the practice. Many times in medical offices date-sensitive information is not entered into MediSoft on the same day that the event or transaction occurred. For example, Friday's office visits may not be entered into MediSoft until Monday. If the MediSoft and Windows dates are not changed to Friday's date before entering the data, all the information entered on Monday will be associated with Monday's date. For this reason, it is important to know how to change the MediSoft Program Date and the Windows System Date.

The following steps are used to change the MediSoft Program Date:

1. Click Set Program Date on the File menu, or click the date displayed on the Status bar. A pop-up calendar is displayed.

2. Click the desired month on the Month drop-down list.

3. Select the desired year by clicking the counter button next to the year.

4. Select the desired date by clicking on that date in the calendar.

5. To save the changes, press Enter or click the green Checkmark button just to the left of the month field.

6. To exit the pop-up calendar without saving the date change, click the red Cancel button.

The following steps are used to change the Windows System Date:

1. Double-click the time displayed on the taskbar (Clock button). The Date/Time Properties dialog box is displayed.

2. Click the desired month on the Month drop-down list.

3. Select the desired year by clicking the counter buttons next to the year. The top button moves ahead; the bottom button moves back.

4. Select the desired date by clicking on that date in the calendar.

5. Click the OK button.

6. To exit the Date/Time Properties dialog box without saving the date change, click the Cancel button.

MMDDYY format a specific way in which dates must be keyed, in which "MM" stands for month, "DD" stands for day, and "YY" stands for year.

MMDDCCYY format a specific way in which dates must be keyed, in which "MM" stands for month, "DD" stands for day, "CCYY" stands for year (using four digits).

In MediSoft dialog boxes, most dates are entered either in the **MMDDYY format** or the **MMDDCCYY format**. The MMDDYY format is a specific way in which dates must be keyed. "MM" stands for the month, "DD" stands for the day, and "YY" stands for the year. Each date must contain two digits, and no punctuation can be used. For example, the date of February 1, 1999, would be keyed as "020199." In other dialog boxes, dates are entered in the MMDDCCYY format. In this format, the month and day are entered as two digits, but the year is entered as four digits. Using the example just mentioned, February 1, 1999, would be keyed as "02011999."

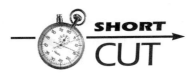

In most MediSoft dialog boxes, dates can be keyed in the text boxes or selected from a pop-up calendar. When the Pop-up Calendar button (see Figure 4-16) is clicked, a small calendar appears on the screen. The current date appears highlighted. To select a different date, the desired month and year are selected from drop-down lists. The day is selected by clicking the Day box on the calendar itself. Pressing the Enter key saves the data, as does clicking the green Checkmark button. Clicking the red Cancel button closes the pop-up calendar without saving any changes.

Figure 4-16 Pop-up Calendar button.

Exercise 4-4

Practice entering information and correcting errors.

MediSoft Program Date: November 17, 2003

Windows System Date: November 17, 2003

1. Click the Activities menu.

2. Click Enter Transactions.

3. Click the triangle button in the Chart box. The Chart drop-down list is displayed (see Figure 4-17).

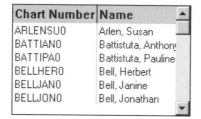

Chart Number	Name
ARLENSUO	Arlen, Susan
BATTIANO	Battistuta, Anthony
BATTIPAO	Battistuta, Pauline
BELLHERO	Bell, Herbert
BELLJANO	Bell, Janine
BELLJONO	Bell, Jonathan

Figure 4-17 Chart drop-down list.

4. To select James Smith, key the first three letters of his chart number (SMITHJAØ): *SMI*

   Notice that when the "S" was keyed, the system went to the entry for the first patient whose chart number begins with "S," in this case James Smith.

5. Press the Enter key.

6. Click the Edit button.

7. Click the Pop-up Calendar button that is next to the first Dates box. Click 21 on the calendar to change the day to May 21. Press the Enter key.

8. Click the second Dates text box. Notice that the system automatically changes the entry to match the date in the first Dates box.

9. Look at the Amount box, where "125.00" is displayed.

10. Click the Procedure box. Then key *99203*. The system highlights the procedure on the drop-down list.

11. Press the Enter key.

12. Look at the Amount box again. The charge associated with the new procedure code, "200.00," is displayed. The system automatically changes the entry in the Amount box to match the entry in the Procedure box (see Figure 4-18).

13. Change the entry in the Amount box from 200.00 to 250.00 by dragging to select the 200.00 and keying *250* and pressing the Enter key. The amount displayed changes to 250.00. Notice how the system automatically adds the decimal point.

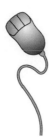

14. Press the Tab key repeatedly and watch as the cursor moves from box to box.

15. Exit the Transaction Entry dialog box without saving these changes. To do this, click the Cancel button at the right side of the dialog box that displays a red "X."

16. You are now back at the main Transaction Entry dialog box. To close this dialog box, click the Close button.

Pop-up Calendar buttons

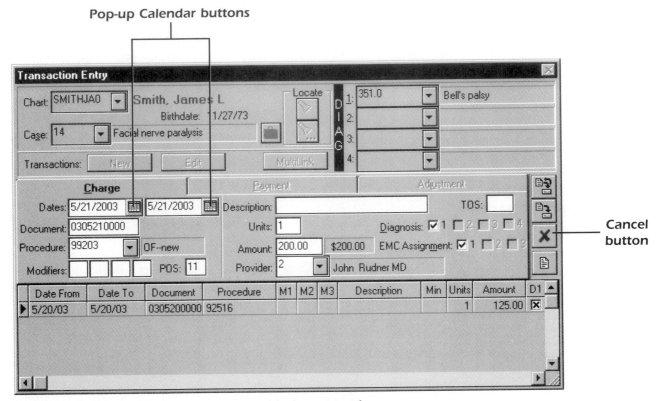

Cancel button

Figure 4-18 Transaction Entry dialog box with data entered.

SAVING DATA   Information entered into MediSoft is saved by clicking the Save button that appears in most dialog boxes (those in which data is input). In an office setting, data is saved to the computer's hard disk. In this text/workbook, however, all data must be saved to the Working Copy disk in Drive A. This allows each student working with MediSoft to complete the exercises in the text/workbook independently. If one student saved data to the hard disk, the next student would find the data already in the system when attempting to complete the exercises.

DELETING DATA   In some MediSoft dialog boxes, there are buttons for the purpose of deleting data. For example, to delete an insurance carrier, the entry for the carrier is clicked in the Insurance Carrier List dialog box.

Then, the Delete button is clicked. MediSoft will ask for a confirmation before deleting the data. In other dialog boxes, such as the Transaction Entry dialog box, there is no button for deleting data. In this situation, the method for deleting data is less obvious. The entry to be deleted is clicked, and then the right mouse button is clicked. A shortcut menu is displayed that contains an option to delete the transaction. Again, MediSoft will ask for confirmation before deleting the data.

BACKING UP DATA

backup data a copy of data files at a specific point in time that can be used to restore data to the system.

Data is periodically saved on removable magnetic media, such as diskettes or tapes, through a process known as backing up. **Backup data** is a copy of data files made at a specific point in time that can be used to restore data to the system. Backups are performed on a regular schedule, determined by the medical practice. Many practices back up data at the end of each day. Backups are only for an office setting. In this text/workbook, the steps required to back up data will be covered, but an actual backup will not be performed.

USING MEDISOFT ONLINE HELP

MediSoft offers two online help features. As discussed in Chapter 3, online help is information provided on the screen, while working on the computer.

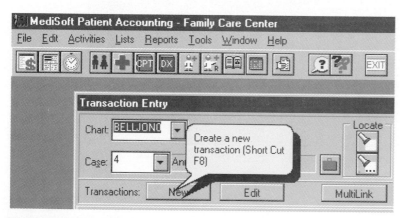

Balloon Help Balloon **help** is information provided through a series of balloons that appear on the screen as the mouse pointer is moved to certain items. The balloons contain text that explains the purpose of the particular item (see Figure 4-19). The text in the balloon also appears on the status bar at the bottom of the screen.

Figure 4-19 Example of balloon help.

balloon help information provided through a series of balloons that appear on the screen.

Help Menu For more detailed online help, MediSoft also has an extensive help feature, accessed through the Help menu.

EXITING MEDISOFT

MediSoft is exited by clicking Exit on the File menu or by clicking the Exit button on the toolbar. To avoid the inconvenience of exiting and restarting MediSoft many times during a day when the computer is needed for a different program, MediSoft can be made temporarily inactive by using the Minimize button, the first of the three small buttons displayed in the upper-right corner of the window. (See Chapter 3 for more information on the Minimize button.) MediSoft can be reactivated at any time by clicking the MediSoft button on the Windows 95 taskbar (see Figure 4-20).

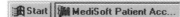

Start | **MediSoft Patient Acc...**   10:34 AM

Figure 4-20 Sample Windows 95 taskbar with MediSoft button.

Exercise 4-5

Practice using MediSoft's Help menu feature.

1. Click the Help menu.

2. Click Table of Contents. MediSoft displays a list of topics for which help is available.

3. Click Diagnosis Entry. Information on entering diagnosis codes is displayed.

4. Print the information by clicking the Print button. The Print dialog box is displayed.

5. Click the OK button to print.

6. To exit Help, click File on the Help menu bar. Then click Exit.

Exercise 4-6

Practice using Balloon help.

1. Click the Activities menu.

2. Click Enter Transactions.

3. Slowly move the mouse pointer over the Chart box. A balloon is displayed with the hint "Enter the chart number here. Press F8 to add a new patient or F9 to edit an existing patient."

4. Point to the Close button. A balloon is displayed with the hint "Close this window."

5. Close the Transaction Entry dialog box.

6. Click the Exit button on the toolbar to exit MediSoft.

CHAPTER REVIEW

USING TERMINOLOGY

Match the terms on the left with the definitions on the right.

_____ **1.** backup data

_____ **2.** balloon help

_____ **3.** MMDDYY format

_____ **4.** MMDDCCYY format

_____ **5.** transactions

a. Help provided through a series of balloons that appear on the screen as the cursor moves to certain items.

b. A way in which dates must be keyed, in which "MM" stands for the month, "DD" stands for the day, and "YY" stands for the year.

c. In MediSoft, charges, payments, and adjustments.

d. A way in which dates must be keyed, in which "MM" stands for the month, "DD" stands for the day, "CCYY" stands for the year (using four digits).

e. A copy of data files made at a specific point in time that can be used to restore data to the system.

CHECKING YOUR UNDERSTANDING

Answer the questions below in the space provided.

6. Describe two ways of issuing a command in MediSoft.

_____

_____

7. What are two ways data are entered in a box?

_____

_____

8. What two types of online help are available in MediSoft?

_____

_____

9. Which menu provides access to Office Hours, MediSoft's scheduling feature?

_____

_____

10. What is the purpose of the buttons on the toolbar?

_____

_____

11. What are the formats for entering dates in MediSoft?

_____

_____

12. Describe two ways of exiting MediSoft.

_____

_____

APPLYING KNOWLEDGE

13. Use MediSoft's Help menu to look up information on the following topics:

- How to use the help feature
- How to print lists from the MediSoft database

AT THE COMPUTER

Answer the following questions at the computer:

14. How many options are there in the Reports menu?

_____

15. What is the first choice on the Lists menu?

_____

16. List the options on the Activities menu.

_____

17. Set the MediSoft Program Date to December 1, 2003. Set the Windows System Date to December 1, 2003.

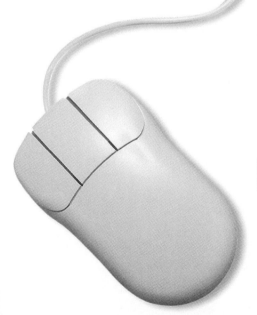

5 Recording Patient Information

WHAT YOU NEED TO KNOW

To use this chapter, you need to know how to:
◆ Start MediSoft.
◆ Move around the MediSoft menus.
◆ Use the MediSoft toolbar.
◆ Enter and edit data in MediSoft.
◆ Exit MediSoft.

OBJECTIVES

In this chapter, you will learn how to:
◆ Use the MediSoft Search feature.
◆ Assign a chart number to a new patient.
◆ Enter personal and employer information on a new patient.
◆ Locate and change information on an established patient.

KEY TERMS

chart number
guarantor

HOW PATIENT INFORMATION IS ORGANIZED IN MEDISOFT

**Patient List
shortcut button.**

Patient information is accessed through the Patient List dialog box. The Patient List dialog box is displayed when Patients/Guarantors and Cases is clicked on the Lists menu or when the corresponding shortcut button is clicked on the toolbar (see left margin).

The Patient List dialog box (see Figure 5-1) is divided into two primary sections. The left side of the window displays information about patients, and the right side of the window contains information about cases. Cases are covered in Chapter 6. At the top right side of the Patient List dialog box, there are two radio buttons: Patient and Case. When the Patient radio button is clicked, the left side of the window becomes active. Correspondingly, when the Case radio button is clicked, the right side of the window becomes active. The command buttons at the bottom of the dialog box vary, depending on which side of the window is active.

The Patient window contains the following data: Chart Number, Name, Date of Birth, Social Security Number, Patient ID #2, Patient Type, Phone 1, Provider, and Last Name. There is not enough room in the Patient window to display all this information, so only a portion is visible at one time. To view the rest of the patient information, it is necessary to use the scroll bars (see Figure 5-2). Scrolling to the right displays information in the additional columns, including Social Security Number, Patient ID #2, and so on. Scrolling down the Patient window displays additional chart numbers and patient names. (Please refer to Chapter 3 for more information on scrolling.) The command buttons at the bottom of the screen include: Edit Patient, New Patient, Delete Patient, and Close.

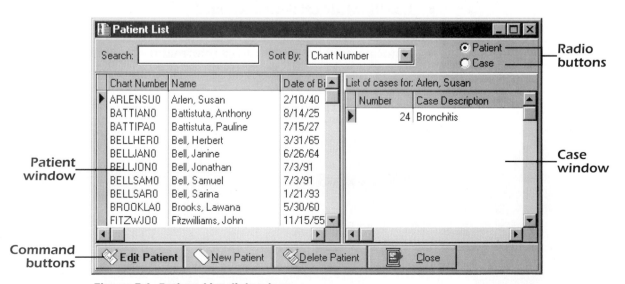

Figure 5-1 Patient List dialog box.

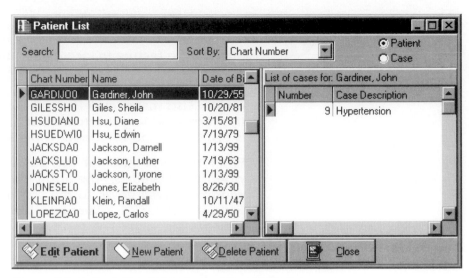

Figure 5-2 Patient List dialog box with scroll bar in use.

SEARCHING FOR PATIENT INFORMATION

When patients come to a medical practice for the first time, they fill out a patient information form. The information on this form needs to be entered into the MediSoft patient/guarantor database before any insurance claims can be submitted. However, before information on a patient is entered into the system, it is important to search the database to be certain that the patient does not already exist in the database.

MediSoft's Search feature is used to look for information on patients, insurance carriers, diagnosis codes, and procedure codes, as well as the names and addresses of employers, and providers. Searches for information on patients are conducted using the Search box in the upper-left corner of the Patient List dialog box (see Figure 5-3).

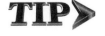

Figure 5-3 Search box.

In a search, MediSoft locates the name or number that most closely matches the letters and/or numbers entered in the Search box. For example, if the letters "SMI" are entered in the Search box, MediSoft will match the first patient with a last name beginning with the letters "SMI." The Search box for patients can contain up to seven letters, including spaces.

TIP ▶ It does not matter whether capital letters or lowercase letters are entered in the Search box. For example, keying "SMITH," "Smith," or "smith" will all locate the first patient in the database with the last name of Smith.

Exercise 5-1

Use the Search feature to locate information on James Smolowski.

1. **Start MediSoft.**

2. **On the Lists menu, click Patients/Guarantors and Cases or click the corresponding shortcut button. The Patient List dialog box is displayed, and the cursor is blinking in the Search box.**

3. **Enter the first letter of the patient's last name. Notice that when you keyed "S," the arrow on the left side of the Patient window moved down to the first patient whose name begins with the letter "S," James L. Smith. Continue entering the patient's last name. As soon as you key the next two letters, "mo," the arrow points to James Smolowski. Smolowski is the only patient whose name begins with the letters "Smo."**

4. **Click the Close button to exit the Patient List dialog box.**

ENTERING NEW PATIENT INFORMATION

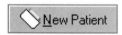

New Patient button.

Information on a new patient is entered in MediSoft by clicking the New Patient button at the bottom of the Patient List dialog box (see left margin). This action opens the Patient/Guarantor dialog box (see Figure 5-4). The Patient/Guarantor dialog box contains two tabs: the Name, Address tab and the Other Information tab.

Name, Address tab

Other Information tab

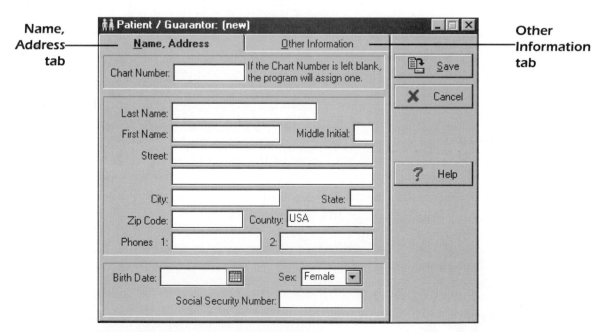

Figure 5-4 Patient/Guarantor dialog box.

NAME, ADDRESS TAB

The Name, Address tab is where basic patient information is entered.

Chart Number

chart number *a unique number that identifies a patient.*

The **chart number** is a unique number that identifies a patient. In MediSoft, a chart number links together all the information about a patient that is stored in the different databases, such as name, address, charges, insurance claims, and so on. Each patient is assigned an eight-character chart number. If the chart number box for a patient is left blank, the system will assign a chart number.

Medical practices may use different methods for assigning chart numbers, although these general guidelines must be followed:

◆ The chart number must start with a letter but can contain a combination of letters and numbers.

◆ No special characters, such as hyphens, periods, or spaces, are allowed.

◆ No two chart numbers can be the same.

For the purposes of this text/workbook, the following method will be used for assigning chart numbers:

◆ The first five characters of the chart number are the first five letters of a patient's last name. If the patient's last name is less than five characters, complete the first five letters with the beginning letters of the patient's first name.

◆ The next two characters are usually the first two letters of a patient's first name. (In a case in which the first two letters of the first name are used to complete the first five letters due to a short last name, the next two letters of the patient's first name are used.)

◆ The last character is always a zero, displayed in this text/workbook with the symbol "Ø."

For example, the chart number for John Fitzwilliams would begin with the first five letters of his last name (FITZW), followed by the first two characters of his first name (JO), followed by a zero (Ø). John's complete chart number would be FITZWJOØ. Following the same rules, John's daughter Sarah would have a chart number of FITZWSAØ.

Exercise 5-2

Create a chart number for each of these patients.

Albert Wong _____

Jessica Sypkowski _____

John James _____

Personal Data

In addition to the chart number, personal information about a patient is entered in the Name, Address tab.

Name, Address, and Phone Numbers   The boxes for name, address, and phone numbers contain basic information about a patient. There are two boxes for phones: the one on the left (1) is for the phone number; the one on the right (2) is for the fax number. If there is no fax number, this box is left blank or an alternate phone number is listed. Phone numbers and fax numbers must be entered without parentheses or hyphens.

Birth Date   The patient's birth date is entered in the Birth Date box using the MMDDCCYY format.

Sex   This drop-down list contains choices for the patient's gender, male or female.

Social Security Number   The nine-digit Social Security Number should be entered with hyphens; however, the system will accept the number if entered without them.

OTHER INFORMATION TAB

The Other Information tab within the Patient/Guarantor dialog box contains facts about a patient's employment and other miscellaneous information (see Figure 5-5).

Type   The Type drop-down list is used to designate whether, for billing purposes, an individual is a patient or guarantor (see Figure 5-6). A **guarantor** is someone who is responsible for insurance and payment. If the individual has insurance, the guarantor is the policyholder. In this context, a patient is an individual who has insurance coverage through someone else. For example, children are typically patients and not guarantors; they are covered under their parents' insurance policy.

guarantor a person responsible for insurance and payment.

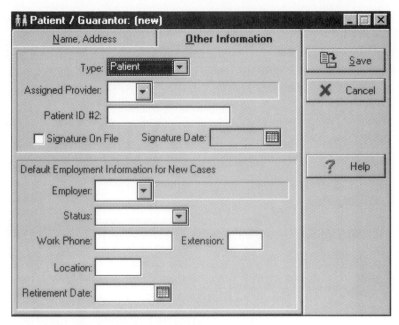

Figure 5-5 Other Information tab.

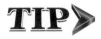 **TIP** A guarantor is not always a patient of the practice. However, information about the guarantor must still be entered into MediSoft if the patient is to receive insurance coverage under the guarantor's policy. For example, children are typically covered by one of their parents' insurance policies. Due to a divorce or other circumstance, both parents may not go to the same physician. In this example, the child is a patient of the practice, but the parent who is the guarantor is a patient of a different medical practice. In this type of situation, the parent is entered as a guarantor in the Type box in the Other Information tab of

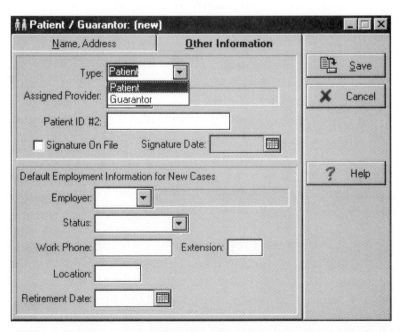

Figure 5-6 Other Information tab with Type drop-down list displayed.

the Patient/Guarantor dialog box. Even though the parent is not a patient of the practice, information about the parent is still entered by clicking the New Patient button in the Patient List dialog box. Then, the child is entered in a separate new Patient/Guarantor dialog box and listed as a patient in the Type box in the Other Information tab.

Assigned Provider   The Assigned Provider drop-down list contains codes assigned to the doctors in the practice (see Figure 5-7). The code for the specific doctor who provides care to this patient is selected.

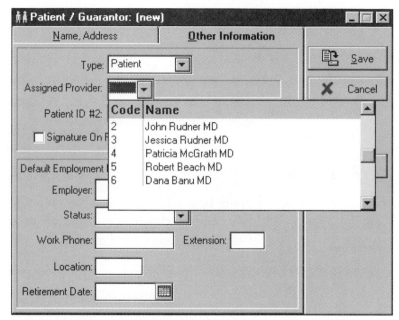

Figure 5-7 Other Information tab with Assigned Provider drop-down list displayed.

Patient ID #2   The Patient ID #2 box is used by some medical practices as a second identification system in addition to chart numbers.

Signature on File   A check mark in the Signature on File check box means that the patient's signature is on file for the purpose of submitting insurance claims.

Signature Date   The date keyed in the Signature Date box is the date the patient signed the insurance release form.

Employer   The code for the patient's employer is selected from the drop-down list of employers that are in the database (see Figure 5-8). If the patient's employer is not in the database, this information must be entered before the code can be selected. (This process is described later in the chapter.)

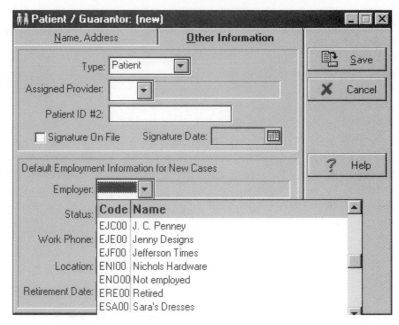

Figure 5-8 Other Information tab with Employer drop-down list displayed.

Status   The Status drop-down list displays the following choices for the patient's employment status: Not employed, Full time, Part time, Retired, or Unknown (see Figure 5-9).

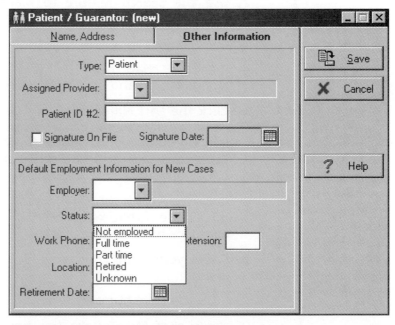

Figure 5-9 Other Information tab with Status drop-down list displayed.

Work Phone and Extension   Work phone numbers should be entered without parentheses or hyphens.

Location Some companies have multiple site locations. If the patient supplies information on the specific company location, it is entered in this box.

Retirement Date The Retirement Date box is only filled in if the patient is already retired. Retirement dates should be entered in the MMDDCCYY format.

When all the fields in the Name, Address tab and the Other Information tab have been filled in, entries should be checked for accuracy. If any of the information needs to be changed, it can easily be corrected. Once the information has been checked and any necessary corrections made, data is saved by clicking the Save button.

Exercise 5-3

Using Source Document 1, complete the Patient/Guarantor dialog box for Hiro Tanaka, a new patient of Dr. Yan's.

MediSoft Program Date: August 9, 2003

Windows System Date: August 9, 2003

1. On the Lists menu, click Patients/Guarantors and Cases, or, click the corresponding shortcut button on the toolbar.

2. Use the Search feature to make sure Hiro Tanaka is not already in the patient database.

3. Click the New Patient button.

4. Create a chart number for this patient. Click the Chart Number box, and enter the chart number.

5. Click the Last Name box, and fill in the patient information. Fill in the rest of the boxes on the Name, Address tab, pressing the Tab key to move from box to box. (Note: Since Tanaka's employer is not in the database, leave the employer boxes blank for now.)

6. Click the Other Information tab, and fill in the appropriate boxes. (Be sure to select an Assigned Provider, or subsequent exercises in this chapter will not work.)

7. Check your entries for accuracy, and make corrections if necessary.

8. Click the Save button to save the data on Ms. Tanaka.

9. Verify that Ms. Tanaka has been added to the list in the Patient List dialog box.

10. Close the Patient List dialog box.

ADDING AN EMPLOYER TO THE ADDRESS LIST

If the patient's employer does not appear on the Employer drop-down list in the Other Information tab, it must be entered through the Addresses command on the Lists menu. When the Addresses command is clicked, the Address List dialog box is displayed (see Figure 5-10). Clicking the New button at the bottom of the Address List dialog box displays the Address dialog box (see Figure 5-11).

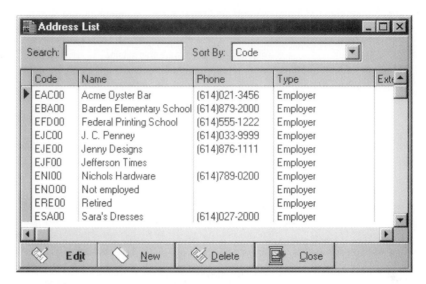

Figure 5-10 Address List dialog box.

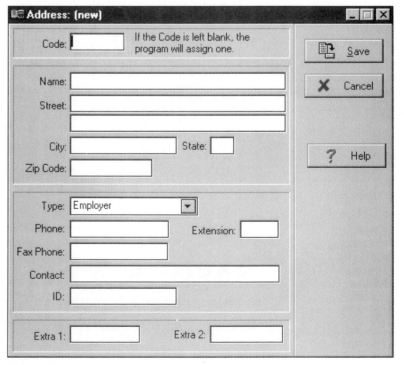

Figure 5-11 Address dialog box.

The Address dialog box contains the following boxes:

Code   The code for an employer should begin with the letter "E," to indicate that this is an employer. Codes can be a combination of letters and numbers, up to a maximum of five characters. If a code is not assigned, the system will assign one.

Name and Address   The employer's name is entered in the Name box. This field allows up to 30 characters. The employer's street, city, state (two characters only), and ZIP Code are entered in the boxes provided.

Type   The Type drop-down list displays a list of kinds of addresses: Attorney, Employer, Facility, Laboratory, Miscellaneous, and Referral Source. For example, when the address being entered is that of an employer, "Employer" would be selected.

Phone, Extension, Fax Phone   In the Phone box, the employer's phone number is entered, without parentheses or hyphens. If there is an extension, it is entered in the Extension box. The employer's fax number is entered in the Fax Phone box, also without parentheses or hyphens.

Contact   The Contact box is used to enter the name of an individual at the place of employment. If there is no contact person, the box is left blank.

ID   If there is an identification number for the employer, it is entered in the ID box.

Extra 1, Extra 2   The Extra 1 and Extra 2 boxes are available to keep track of any additional information that needs to be recorded and stored for future reference.

When all the information on the employer has been entered, it is saved by clicking the Save button.

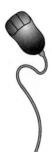

Exercise 5-4

Practice entering information on an employer.

MediSoft Program Date: August 9, 2003

Windows System Date: August 9, 2003

1. **Click Addresses on the Lists menu. The Address List dialog box is displayed.**

2. Click the **New** button at the bottom of the dialog box. The Address dialog box is displayed.

3. In the Code box, key *EMCØØ* for McCray Manufacturing, Inc. ("E" for employer, followed by the first two letters of the employer's name, followed by two zeros.) Press the Tab key.

4. Key *McCray Manufacturing Inc* in the Name box. Press the Tab key.

5. In the Street box, key *1311 Kings Highway*. Press the Tab key twice.

6. Key *Stephenson* in the City box. Press the Tab key.

7. Key *OH* in the State box. Press the Tab key.

8. Key *60089* in the ZIP Code box. Press the Tab key.

9. Verify that "Employer" is displayed in the Type box. If it is not, click Employer in the drop-down list and press the Tab key.

10. Key *6145550000* in the Phone box. Press the Tab key.

11. Since there is no extension or fax phone listed, leave the corresponding boxes blank.

12. Since there is no information on a contact, an ID, or any extra information, leave the corresponding boxes blank.

13. Click the **Save** button to store the information you have entered.

14. Click the **Close** button to exit the Address List dialog box.

EDITING INFORMATION ON AN ESTABLISHED PATIENT

From time to time, established patients notify the practice that they have moved, changed jobs or insurance carriers, and so on. When this happens, information needs to be updated in MediSoft's patient/guarantor database. The process of changing information on an established patient is similar to that of entering information on a new patient. The patient information is accessed through the Patient List dialog box. Then the Patients/Guarantors and Cases command is selected from the Lists menu. A search is usually performed first to locate the name or chart number of the patient whose record needs to be updated. Data can be edited either by pressing the Enter key or by clicking the Edit Patient button at the bottom of the dialog box. This displays the Patient/Guarantor dialog box, where changes can be made. Clicking the Save button stores the changes.

Exercise 5-5

Practice searching for and editing information on Hiro Tanaka.

MediSoft Program Date: August 9, 2003

Windows System Date: August 9, 2003

1. Open the Patient List dialog box.

2. Search for Hiro Tanaka by entering her chart number, TANAKHIØ. When the search is done, the selection arrow should be pointing to Tanaka, Hiro.

3. Click the Edit Patient button.

4. Click the Other Information tab.

5. Click the triangle button in the employer box. Click McCray Manufacturing Inc, on the drop-down list.

6. In the Work Phone box, delete the phone number that appears and key *6145551001*.

7. Click the Save button to store the information you have entered.

8. Close the Patient List dialog box.

9. Exit MediSoft.

CHAPTER REVIEW

USING TERMINOLOGY

Define the terms in the space provided.

1. chart number

_____

_____

2. guarantor

_____

_____

CHECKING YOUR UNDERSTANDING

Answer the questions below in the space provided.

3. To search for Paul Ramos, can you key either "Paul" or "Ramos"? Explain.

_____

_____

4. Create a chart number for a patient with the name of William Burroughs.

_____

_____

5. Sam Wu has no insurance of his own but is covered by his wife's insurance policy. How would you indicate this in the Patient/Guarantor dialog box?

_____

_____

6. A patient's address is 11 West Main Street, Anytown, WI 55555. What would you enter in the City box located within the Patient/Guarantor dialog box?

_____

_____

7. How would you enter the Social Security Number 123-45-6789?

_____

CHAPTER REVIEW

APPLYING KNOWLEDGE

Answer the following question in the space provided.

8. Jane Taylor-Burke comes to the office. She thinks she saw Dr. Yan a few years ago for a flu shot, but she is not sure. You need to decide whether to enter Ms. Taylor-Burke as a new patient in the MediSoft database. What should you do?

_____

_____

_____

_____

AT THE COMPUTER

Answer the following questions at the computer:

9. How many patients in the database have the last name of Smith?

_____

10. List the name of the patient that is found when you search for the letters "JO"?

_____

11. What is Li Y Wong's chart number?

_____

12. In the Patient List dialog box, search for information on Leila Patterson. What steps did you take to find the information?

_____

_____

_____

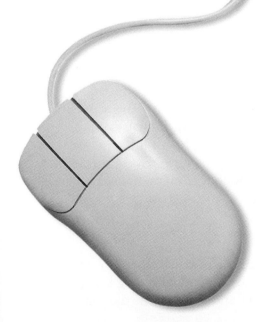

CHAPTER

6 Working with Cases

OBJECTIVES

In this chapter, you will learn how to:

- ◆ Set up a new case.
- ◆ Enter information on a patient's insurance policy.
- ◆ Enter information on an accident or illness.
- ◆ Enter information on a patient's diagnosis.
- ◆ Add a new referring provider to the database.
- ◆ Add a new insurance carrier to the database.
- ◆ Edit information in an existing case.
- ◆ Close a case.
- ◆ Delete a case.

KEY TERMS

capitated plan   record of treatment and progress
cases   referring provider
chart   sponsor
Medigap

WHAT IS A CASE?

Cases are groupings of transactions for visits to a physician's office, organized around a condition. When a patient comes for treatment, a case is created.

Cases are set up to contain the transactions that relate to a particular condition. For example, all treatments and procedures for bronchial asthma would be stored in a case called "Bronchial asthma." Services performed and charges for those services are entered in the system and linked to the bronchial asthma case.

WHEN TO SET UP A NEW CASE

New cases should be set up each time a patient comes to see the physician for a new condition or when there is a change in the provider or insurance carrier. For example, suppose a patient has been seeing a physician regularly for treatment of bronchial asthma. All the transactions for this treatment would be contained in one case. Then suppose the patient has an accident at work and comes in for treatment of a sprained ankle. A new case would be set up in MediSoft for the sprained-ankle treatments. The sprained ankle is a new condition.

When a patient changes insurance carriers, a new case should be set up, even if the same condition is being treated under the new carrier. This makes it easier to submit insurance claims to the appropriate carrier. Transactions that took place while the previous policy was in effect must be submitted under that policy. Transactions that occur after the change in policies must be submitted to the new carrier. By opening a new case, transactions for the two insurance carriers can be kept separate. The information needed to submit claims to the previous carrier is still intact, while information for claims under the new policy is current.

It is common for patients to have more than one case open at any one time. For example, in the example just mentioned, the patient would have a bronchial asthma case and a sprained-ankle case open at the same time. While the patient is being treated for the ankle injury, the bronchial asthma treatment is continuing. Some cases are for chronic conditions and remain open a long time. Other cases, such as a case for treatment of influenza NOS, may be of short duration. Cases are closed when the patient is no longer being treated for the condition, when the insurance policy in a case is no longer in effect, or when the patient leaves the practice.

CASE COMMAND BUTTONS

In MediSoft, cases are created, edited, and deleted from within the Patient List dialog box (see Figure 6-1). The Patient List dialog box is accessed by choosing Patients/Guarantors and Cases from the Lists

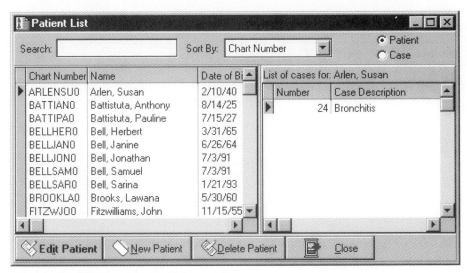

Figure 6-1 Patient List dialog box.

menu. When the Case radio button in the Patient List dialog box is clicked, the following command buttons appear at the bottom of the Patient List dialog box: Edit Case, New Case, Delete Case, Copy Case, and Close (see Figure 6-2).

Case command buttons —

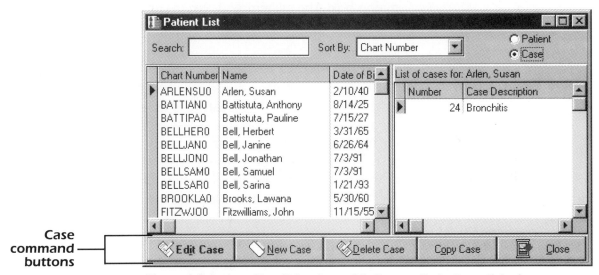

Figure 6-2 Patient List dialog box with Case radio button clicked.

Edit Case Button

The Edit Case button is used to add, delete, or change information in an existing case. When the Edit Case button is clicked, the Case dialog box is displayed. Information to be updated on the case is contained in nine different tabs. For example, if a patient changes insurance carriers, information needs to be updated in the Policy 1, 2, or 3 tabs. The only item in the Case dialog box that cannot be changed is the Case Number. All other boxes are edited by moving the cursor to the box and making the change, whether this means rekeying, selecting and deselecting a check box, or clicking a different option on a drop-down list.

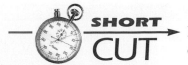 In the Patient List dialog box, cases can also be edited by double-clicking the desired case number/description.

New Case

The New Case button creates a new case.

Delete Case

The Delete Case button deletes a case from the system. The Delete Case button should be used with caution; once deleted, information cannot be retrieved. Cases should be deleted only when it is definite that the patient's records will never be needed again. Medical offices usually have policies about when a patient's records are deleted. For example, a medical office may delete the billing records of a deceased patient 12 months after the death.

Cases are deleted in the Patient List dialog box. With the Case radio button clicked, the specific case to be deleted is selected by clicking the line that displays the case number and description. The case is then deleted by clicking the Delete Case button at the bottom of the dialog box. The system will ask, "Are you sure you want to delete this case?" Clicking the Yes button deletes the case from the system.

Copy Case

The Copy Case button copies all the information from an existing case into a new case. This feature is useful when creating a new case for a patient who already has a case in the system. Rather than reenter the information in all nine tabs, the information in the existing case is copied into a new case. Then the information that needs to be changed can be edited to reflect the data relevant to the new case. The information that remains the same can be left as is.

Close

The Close button closes the Patient List dialog box.

Save

After the information in all nine tabs has been checked for accuracy and edited as necessary, the case must be saved. Data recorded in the Case dialog box is stored by clicking the Save button on the right side of the Case dialog box. Clicking the Cancel button exits the Case dialog box without saving the newly entered information. The boxes that had new data entered will clear, and the screen will redisplay the Patient List dialog box.

ENTERING CASE INFORMATION

Clicking the New Case button or the Edit Case button brings up the Case dialog box. Information on a patient is entered in nine different tabs within the Case dialog box:

- Personal
- Account
- Diagnosis
- Policy 1
- Policy 2
- Policy 3
- Condition
- Medicaid and CHAMPUS
- Miscellaneous

chart *a folder that contains all records pertaining to a patient.*

record of treatment and progress *a record containing physician's notes about a patient's condition and diagnosis.*

The information required to complete the nine tabs comes from documents found in a patient's chart. The **chart** is a folder that contains all records pertaining to a patient. The new patient information form supplies basic information such as name and address as well as information about insurance coverage, allergies, whether the condition is related to an accident, and the referral source. The **record of treatment and progress** contains physician's notes about a patient's condition and diagnosis. The superbill is a list of services performed and charges for these procedures.

PERSONAL TAB

The Personal tab contains basic information about a patient and his or her employment (see Figure 6-3).

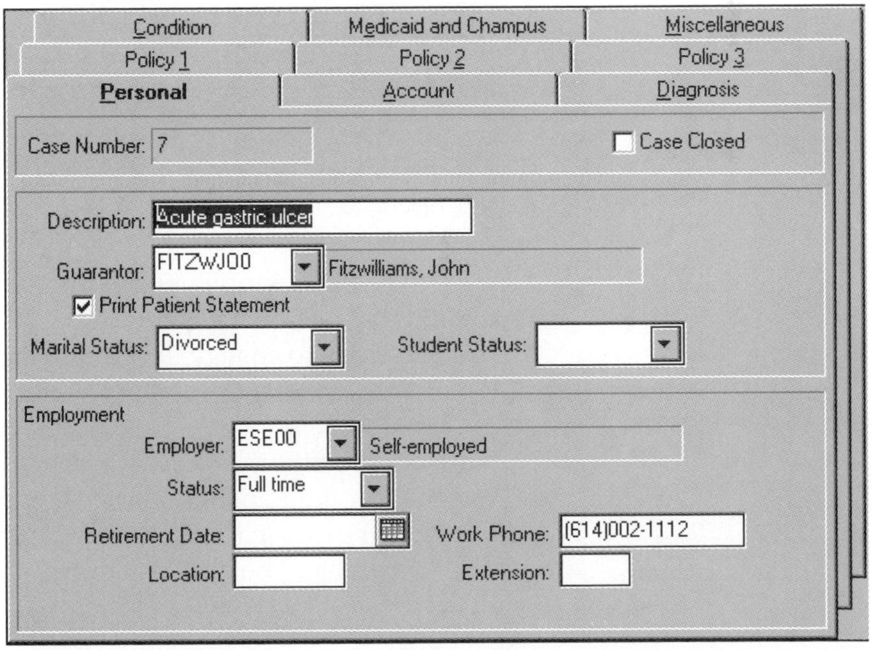

Figure 6-3 Personal tab.

Case Number   The case number is a sequential number assigned by MediSoft. To avoid confusion, case numbers are unique; no two patients ever have the same case number.

Case Closed   A case is marked as closed by placing a check mark in the Case Closed box. At times it is appropriate to close a case. Closing a case indicates that no more data will be entered into the case. When is it appropriate to close a case? Policies vary from practice to practice, but generally cases are closed when a patient changes insurance carriers, has recovered completely from a condition (such as the flu), or is no longer a patient at the practice.

Description   Information entered in the Description box indicates a patient's complaint, or reason for seeing a physician. For example, if a patient comes to see a physician in the practice for an annual physical examination, the Description box would read, "annual physical." Other examples of entries are sore throat, stomach pains, dog bite, accident at work, and so on. A patient's complaint can be found in his or her chart.

Guarantor   The Guarantor box lists the name of the person responsible for paying the bill. The drop-down list contains the chart numbers and names of all potential guarantors in the database.

Print Patient Statement   If this box is checked, a statement for the patient is automatically printed when statements are printed for the practice.

Marital Status   The drop-down list provides the following choices to indicate a patient's marital status: Divorced, Legally separated, Married, Single, Unknown, or Widowed.

Student Status   The Student Status drop-down list is used to indicate whether a patient is a full-time student, a part-time student, or a non-student. If a patient's status is not known, the box should be left blank.

Employer   The Employer box contains the default employer information that has been entered in the Patient/Guarantor dialog box. If it is necessary to change the employer, the default can be overridden by clicking another employer code on the drop-down list.

Status   The Status box lists a patient's employment status as it is recorded in the Patient/Guarantor dialog box. To change the selection that appears in the Status box, another selection is clicked on the drop-down list. The options are Full-time, Not employed, Part-time, Retired, and Unknown.

Retirement Date   The Retirement Date box should be filled in only when a patient is already retired. There are two ways of entering the retirement date. The date can be entered in the Retirement Date box, or can be selected from the calendar that appears when the Pop-up Calendar button at the right of the box is clicked.

Location   If a patient has supplied a specific work location, such as "5th Avenue Branch," it is entered in the Location box.

Work Phone   The Work Phone box contains a patient's work phone number.

Extension   The Extension box lists a patient's work phone extension.

Exercise 6-1

Create a new case for patient Hiro Tanaka, and enter information in the Personal tab. The information needed to complete this exercise is found on Source Document 1.

MediSoft Program Date: August 9, 2003

Windows System Date: August 9, 2003

1. Start MediSoft.

2. On the Lists menu, click Patients/Guarantors and Cases. The Patient List dialog box is displayed.

3. Search for Hiro Tanaka by keying *TAN* in the Search box. The arrow should point to the entry line for Hiro Tanaka.

4. Click the Case radio button to activate the case portion of the Patient List dialog box.

5. Click the New Case button. The dialog box labeled "Case: TANAKHI0 - (new)" is displayed. The Personal tab is the current active tab. Notice that some information is already filled in.

6. Enter Tanaka's reason for seeing the doctor in the Description box.

7. Choose the correct entry for Tanaka's marital status from the drop-down list in the Marital Status box. The Student Status box can be left blank.

8. Notice that the information on Tanaka's employment is already filled in. The system copies the information entered in the Patient/Guarantor dialog box to the case file for you.

9. Check your entries for accuracy.

10. **Click the Save button to save the case information you just entered. The Patient List dialog box redisplays. Notice that the case you just created is listed in the area of the dialog box labeled "List of cases for Tanaka, Hiro."**

11. **Do not close the Patient List dialog box.**

ACCOUNT TAB

The Account tab includes information on a patient's assigned provider, referring provider, referral source, as well as other information that may be used in some medical practices but not others (see Figure 6-4).

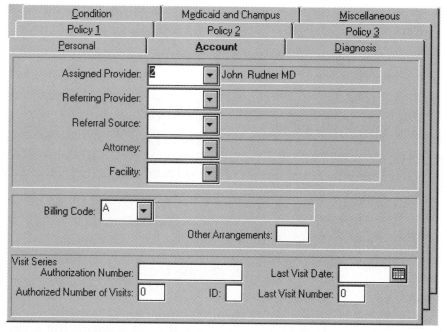

Figure 6-4 Account tab.

Assigned Provider The Assigned Provider box is automatically filled in with the code number and name of the assigned provider listed in the Patient/Guarantor dialog box. The drop-down list provides a complete list of providers in the practice. If necessary, the Assigned Provider selection can be changed by clicking another provider on the list.

referring provider *a physician who recommends that a patient see another specific physician.*

Referring Provider A **referring provider** is a physician who recommends that a patient see another specific physician. The Referring Provider box contains the name of the physician who referred the patient to the practice. The referring provider's name and code are selected from the drop-down list. If the referring provider is not listed on the drop-down list, he or she will need to be added to the Referring Provider list, which is found on the Lists menu. It is not necessary to close the Case dialog box to add a referring provider to the database. When Referring Providers is clicked on the Lists menu, the Referring Provider List dialog box opens in front of the other dialog boxes displayed on the screen. Instructions for adding a referring provider to the database are covered later in this chapter.

Referral Source   If known, the source of a patient's referral is selected from the drop-down list of choices.

Attorney   If a patient has an attorney, the name of the attorney should be selected from the drop-down list. If the attorney is not listed, he or she will need to be added to the system by clicking Addresses on the Lists menu and entering information about the attorney.

Facility   The Facility box lists the place where a patient is receiving treatment. A facility is selected from the drop-down list. When necessary, facilities can be added to the database by clicking Addresses on the Lists menu and entering the necessary information.

Billing Code   The Billing Code box is a one- or two-character box used by some practices to classify and sort patients by insurance carrier, diagnosis, billing cycle, and so on.

Other Arrangements   If a special arrangement is made for billing, it is indicated in the Other Arrangements box.

Visit Series   Information in the Visit Series section of the Account tab is used primarily by psychotherapy practices and chiropractors.

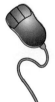

Exercise 6-2

Complete the Account tab for Hiro Tanaka. The information needed to complete this exercise is found on Source Document 1.

MediSoft Program Date: August 9, 2003

Windows System Date: August 9, 2003

1. In the Patient List dialog box, click the line with Hiro Tanaka's name. Then click the Case radio button.

2. Click the Edit Case button to add information to Tanaka's case file. The Case dialog is displayed, with the Personal tab active.

3. Make the Account tab active. The word "Account" should now be displayed in boldfaced type, and the boxes on the Account tab should be visible.

4. Notice that the Assigned Provider box is already filled in with the name of Tanaka's assigned provider, Katherine Yan. The system copies this information from data stored in the Patient/Guarantor dialog box.

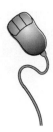

5. Click the name of Tanaka's referring provider on the Referring Provider drop-down list.

6. Check your work for accuracy.

7. Save the changes. The Patient List dialog box is redisplayed.

8. Do not close the Patient List dialog box.

ADDING A REFERRING PROVIDER TO THE DATABASE

If a referring provider is not listed in the Referring Provider drop-down list in the Account tab, he or she will need to be added to the database. To add a referring provider, click Referring Providers on the Lists menu. The Referring Provider List dialog box is then displayed (see Figure 6-5). Clicking the New button brings up the Referring Provider dialog box, which is where information on a new referring provider is entered (see Figure 6-6). The Referring Provider dialog box contains two tabs: Address, and PINs and IDs.

Address Tab

The Address tab includes a provider's name, address, license number, specialty, and Medicare participation status (see Figure 6-7).

Code   The Code box contains a unique identification code assigned to a referring provider. It can be up to five characters. If a code is not entered in the Code box, the system will assign one.

Name, Address, and Phone Numbers   The Last Name, Middle Initial, First Name, Street, City, State, ZIP Code, Phone, and Fax boxes list basic information about a referring provider.

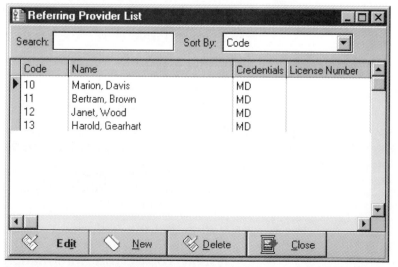

Figure 6-5 Referring Provider List dialog box.

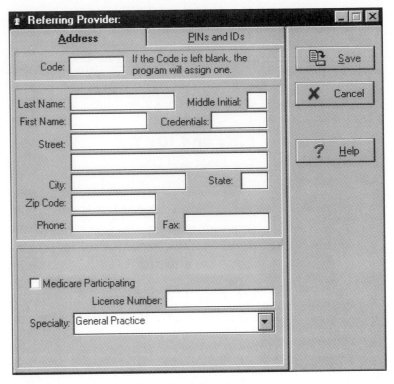

Figure 6-6 Referring Provider dialog box.

Credentials   The Credentials box lists a referring provider's professional credentials, such as MD, DO, PhD, RN, and so on. This box can be up to three characters long.

Medicare Participating   If a referring provider is a participating Medicare provider, the Medicare Participating box is checked.

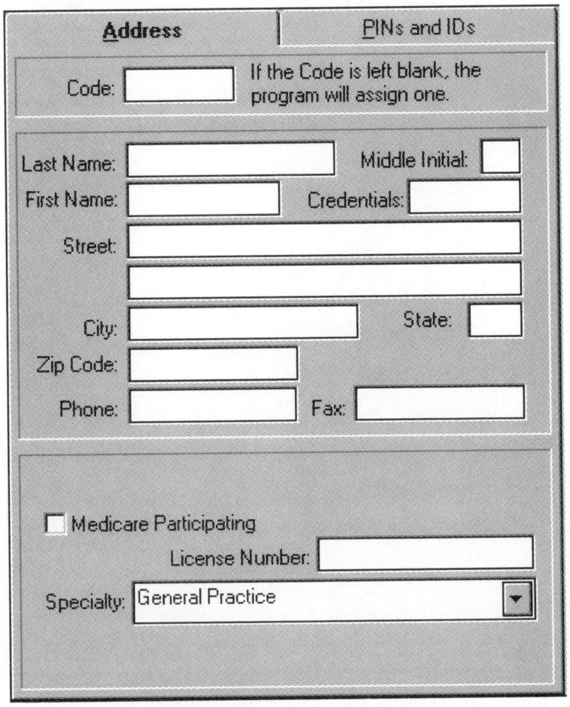

Figure 6-7 Address tab.

License Number   A referring provider's license number is listed in the License Number box.

Specialty   A referring provider's specialty is selected from the corresponding drop-down list. If the specialty is not one of the choices on the list, click the category "All other."

PINs and IDs Tab

The PINs and IDs tab contains identification numbers assigned to a referring provider (see Figure 6-8).

SSN/Federal Tax ID   The SSN/Federal Tax ID box contains a provider's Social Security number or Federal Tax Identification number. If the Federal Tax Identification Number is entered, the box labeled "Federal Tax ID Indicator" should also be checked.

PINs   In the boxes listed, a referring provider's PIN (provider identification number) is entered for each insurance type: Medicare, Medicaid, CHAMPUS, Blue Cross/Shield, Commercial, PPO, and HMO.

Group Number   The Group Number box is where a referring provider's group number is entered. The group number is the identification number for a referring provider's practice.

UPIN   The provider's Unique Physician Identifier Number (UPIN) is entered in the UPIN box.

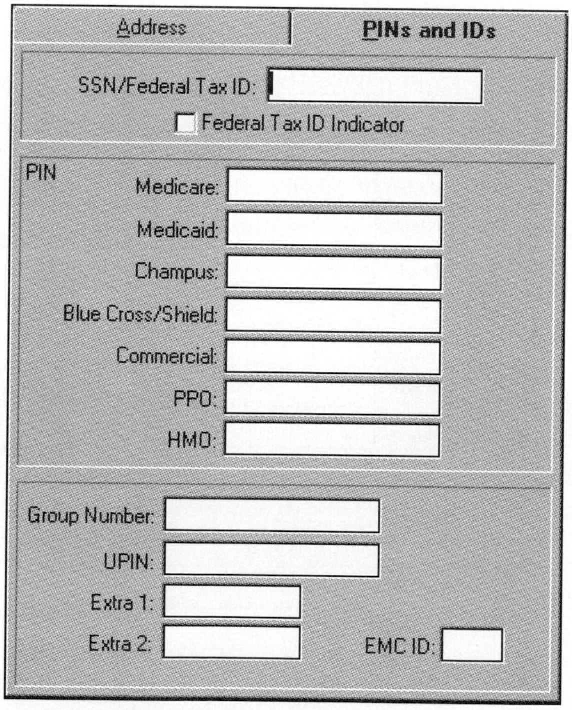

Figure 6-8 PINs and IDs tab.

Extra 1, Extra 2 These boxes can be used to enter any additional information about the referring provider.

EMC ID The EMC ID box contains the identification number assigned to a physician by the EMC clearinghouse.

When all the information on the referring provider has been entered and checked for accuracy, it is saved by clicking the Save button in the Referring Provider dialog box.

DIAGNOSIS TAB The Diagnosis tab contains a patient's diagnosis, information about allergies, and electronic media claim (EMC) notes (see Figure 6-9).

Diagnosis 1 through Diagnosis 4 A patient's diagnosis is selected from the drop-down list of diagnoses. If a patient has more than one diagnosis, the primary diagnosis is entered as Diagnosis 1. Up to four diagnoses can be entered for each case. If there are more than four diagnoses, a new case must be opened.

Allergies and Notes If a patient has allergies or any other special condition that needs to be recorded, it is entered in the Allergies and Notes box.

EMC Notes If a patient's claims require special handling when submitted electronically, notes about the procedure are listed in this box.

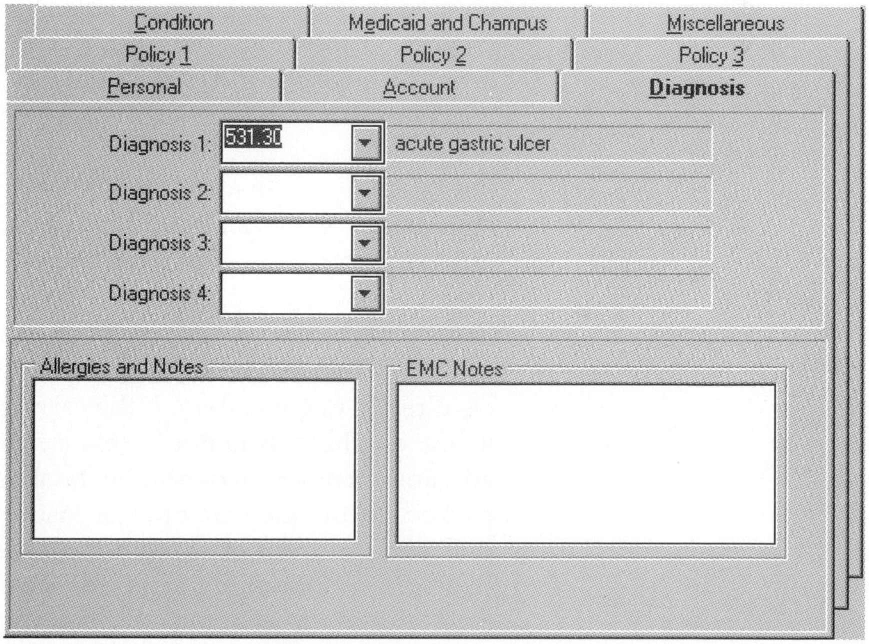

Figure 6-9 Diagnosis tab.

Exercise 6-3

Complete the Diagnosis tab for Hiro Tanaka. The information needed to complete this exercise is found on Source Documents 1 and 4.

MediSoft Program Date: August 9, 2003

Windows System Date: August 9, 2003

1. Edit the case for Hiro Tanaka.

2. Make the Diagnosis tab active.

3. From the list of choices in the drop-down list, select Tanaka's diagnosis.

4. In the Allergies and Notes box, enter information on Tanaka's allergies.

5. Check your work for accuracy.

6. Save the changes. The Patient List dialog box is redisplayed.

7. Do not close the Patient List dialog box.

POLICY 1 TAB The Policy 1 tab is where information about a patient's primary insurance carrier and coverage is recorded (see Figure 6-10).

Insured 1 The Insured 1 box lists the person who is the insured for a particular policy. For example, if the patient is a child covered under a parent's insurance plan, the parent's chart number would be entered in this box. The insured's chart number is selected from the choices on the drop-down list. (If the insured is not a patient of the practice, he or she must be entered as a guarantor in MediSoft and a chart number must be established.)

Relationship to Insured This box describes a patient's relationship to the individual listed in the Insured 1 box. The drop-down list offers the following choices: Child, Other, Self, and Spouse.

Insurance 1 The Insurance 1 box lists the code number and name of the insurance carrier. The drop-down list provides a list of carriers already in the system. If the carrier is not listed, it must be added to the database. It is not necessary to close the Case dialog box to add an insurance carrier to the database. When Insurance Carriers is clicked on the Lists menu, the Insurance Carrier List dialog box is displayed in front of the other dialog boxes shown on the screen. Instructions for adding an insurance carrier to the database are covered later in this chapter.

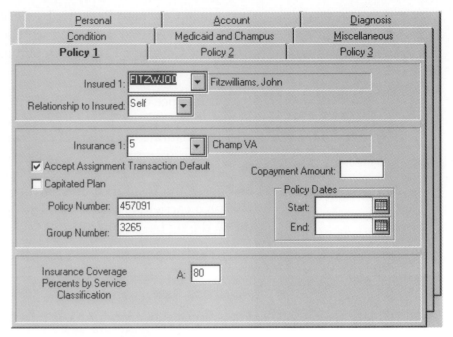

Figure 6-10 Policy 1 tab.

Accept Assignment Transaction Default   For physicians who are participating in an insurance plan, a check mark in the Accept Assignment Transaction Default box indicates that the provider accepts payment directly from the insurance carrier.

Capitated Plan   In a **capitated plan**, payments are made to physicians from managed care companies for patients who select the physician as their primary care provider, regardless of whether they visit the physician or not. A check mark in this box indicates that this insurance plan is capitated.

capitated plan a type of insurance plan in which payments are made to physicians from managed care companies for patients who select the physician as their primary care provider, regardless of whether they visit the physician.

Policy Number   A patient's policy number is entered in the Policy Number box.

Group Number   The group number for a patient's policy is entered in the Group Number box.

Policy Dates—Start/End   The date a patient's insurance policy went into effect is entered in the Policy Dates—Start box. If the date is not known, the date the patient first came to the practice for treatment can be entered. If the policy has ended, such as when the carrier changes or when the coverage expires, the date coverage terminated is entered in the Policy Dates—End box.

Copayment Amount   The dollar amount of a patient's copayment per visit is entered in the Copayment Amount box.

Insurance Coverage Percents by Service Classification   The percentage of fees that an insurance carrier covers is entered in the Insurance Coverage Percents by Service Classification box.

ADDING AN INSURANCE CARRIER TO THE DATABASE

If an insurance carrier is not listed in the Insurance drop-down list in the Policy 1, 2, or 3 tabs, it needs to be added to the database. To add an insurance carrier, click Insurance Carriers on the Lists menu. The Insurance Carrier List dialog box lists all the carriers already in the system (see Figure 6-11). Clicking the New button brings up the Insurance Carrier (new) dialog box, where information on a carrier is entered (see Figure 6-12). The Insurance Carrier (new) dialog box contains three tabs: Address; Options; and EMC, Codes.

Address Tab

The Address tab contains basic information about an insurance carrier (see Figure 6-13).

Code   The code is a unique identification number assigned to an insurance carrier. It can be up to five characters. If a code is not entered in the Code box, the system will assign one.

Name, Address, and Phone Numbers   The Name, Street, City, State, ZIP Code, Phone, Extension, and Fax boxes list basic information about a carrier.

Contact   If there is a specific person at the insurance carrier who is assigned to handle the practice's claims, that person's name is entered in the Contact box.

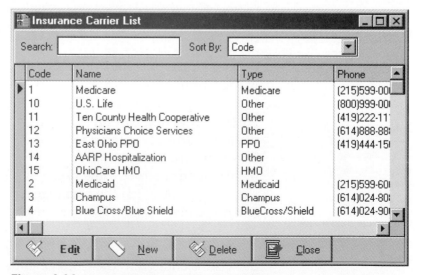

Figure 6-11 Insurance Carrier List dialog box.

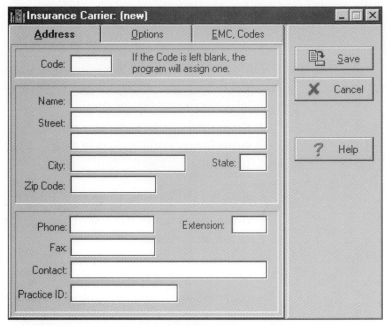

Figure 6-12 Insurance Carrier (new) dialog box.

Practice ID   The Practice ID box lists the identification number assigned to the practice by an insurance carrier.

Options Tab

The Options tab records detailed information about an insurance carrier (see Figure 6-14 on page 104).

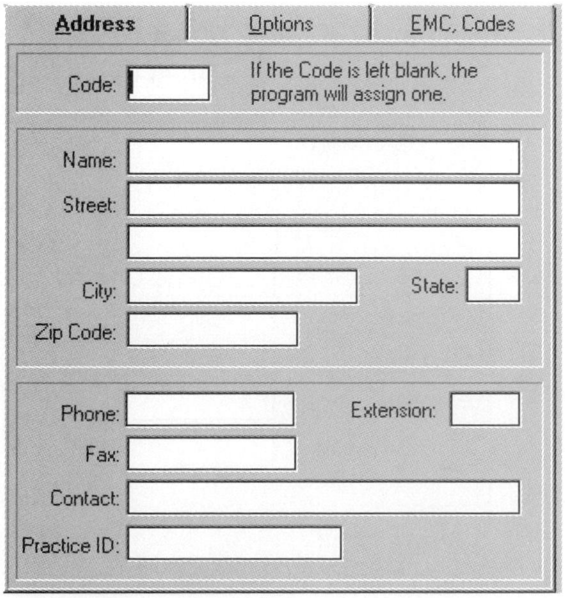

Figure 6-13 Address tab.

Plan Name   The name of the insurance plan is entered in the Plan Name box.

Type   The type of insurance plan is selected from a drop-down list of choices, including Medicare, Blue Cross/Shield, HMO, and so on.

Procedure Code Set   If a practice uses more than one set of procedure codes, enter the code number for the set used by the particular insurance carrier.

Diagnosis Code Set   If a practice uses more than one set of diagnosis codes, enter the code number for the set used by the particular insurance carrier.

Signature on File   The Signature on File box controls whether a patient's signature is printed on an insurance claim form to indicate that he or she has authorized payment to be sent directly to the provider. The choices on the drop-down list are Leave blank, Signature on file, and Print name.

Default Billing Method   The Default Billing Method box indicates whether claims are to be submitted electronically or on paper. For the purposes of this text/workbook, the default method for submitting claims is electronic.

Print PINs on Forms   The Print PINs on Forms box indicates whether the provider name and PINs are to be printed on claim forms.

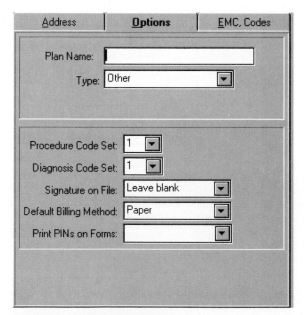

Figure 6-14 Options tab.

EMC, Codes Tab

The third tab in the Insurance Carrier (new) dialog box is the EMC, Codes tab. This tab contains information on electronic media claims (see Figure 6-15).

EMC Receiver   The EMC Receiver box contains the name of the receiver of electronic media claims for a particular insurance carrier.

EMC Payor Number   The payor identification number assigned by the clearinghouse is entered in the EMC Payor Number box.

EMC Sub ID   The EMC Sub ID box contains the sub ID number assigned by the clearinghouse.

EMC Extra 1 and 2   The EMC Extra 1 and EMC Extra 2 boxes can be used to enter additional information about the EMC setup.

NDC Record Code   The record code assigned by the clearinghouse is entered in the NDC (National Data Corporation) Record Code box.

When all the information on an insurance carrier has been entered and checked for accuracy, data is saved by clicking the Save button.

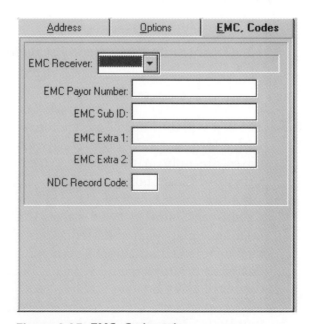

Figure 6-15 EMC, Codes tab.

Exercise 6-4

Complete the Policy 1 tab for Hiro Tanaka. The information needed to complete this exercise is found on Source Document 1.

MediSoft Program Date: August 9, 2003

Windows System Date: August 9, 2003

1. Edit the case for Hiro Tanaka.

2. Make the Policy 1 tab active.

3. Select the chart number and name of the person who should be entered in the Insured 1 box from the list of choices in the Insured 1 box drop-down list.

4. Notice that the Relationship to Insured box already has "Self" entered. If this is correct, do not make any changes. If it is incorrect, make another selection from the drop-down list.

5. Select Tanaka's insurance carrier from the list of choices in the Insurance 1 box.

6. Dr. Yan accepts assignment for this carrier, so click the Accept Assignment Transaction Default box.

7. Enter Tanaka's insurance policy number in the Policy Number box.

8. Enter Tanaka's group number in the Group Number box.

9. In the Policy Dates—Start box, key *08082003* **as the start date of the policy.**

10. Edit the Insurance Coverage Percents by Service Classification box.

11. Check your work for accuracy.

12. Save the changes.

13. Do not close the Patient List dialog box.

POLICY 2 TAB

The boxes in the Policy 2 tab are the same as those in the Policy 1 tab, with a few exceptions. The Copayment Amount and Capitated Plan boxes are only in the Policy 1 tab. Only the Policy 2 tab has a Crossover Claim box (see Figure 6-16).

Crossover Claim   The Crossover Claim box is used to indicate an insurance plan such as a Medigap policy. **Medigap** is a supplementary insurance plan offered by a private insurance company that is designed to supplement Medicare. Because Medicare is the primary carrier, it pays first on a claim and then submits the claim to the Medigap carrier. If the Crossover Claim box is checked, it indicates that Policy 2 is a Medigap plan.

Medigap a supplementary insurance pan offered by a private insurance company that is designed to supplement Medicare.

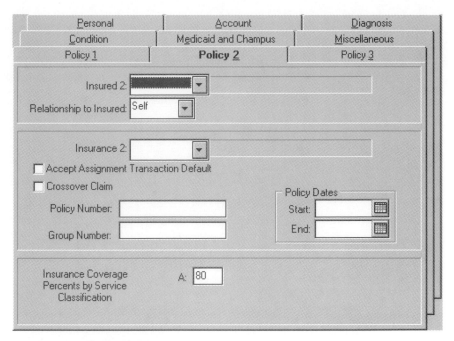

Figure 6-16 Policy 2 tab.

POLICY 3 TAB   The Policy 3 tab does not contain the Copayment Amount, Capitated Plan, and Crossover Claim boxes. Otherwise, the boxes are the same as those in the Policy 1 and Policy 2 tabs (see Figure 6-17).

CONDITION TAB   The Condition tab stores data about a patient's illness, accident, disability, and hospitalization (see Figure 6-18 on page 108). This information is used by insurance carriers to process claims.

Figure 6-17 Policy 3 tab.

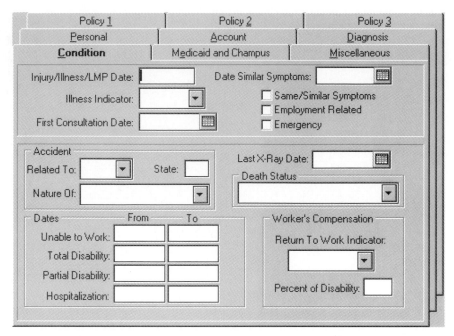

Figure 6-18 Condition tab.

Injury/Illness/LMP Date   The date of a patient's injury, illness, or last menstrual period (LMP) is entered in the Injury/Illness/LMP Date box. (For an illness, the date when the symptom(s) first appeared is entered.)

Illness Indicator   The Illness Indicator box specifies whether a patient's condition is an illness or a last menstrual period, in the case of a pregnancy.

First Consultation Date   The date of a patient's first visit for a particular condition is entered in the First Consultation Date box. The actual date can be entered or the pop-up calendar can be activated and dates selected from the calendar.

Date Similar Symptoms   If a patient has had similar symptoms in the past, enter the date of those symptoms in the Date Similar Symptoms box.

Same/Similar Symptoms   A check mark in the Same/Similar Symptoms box indicates that a patient has had the same or similar symptoms in the past.

Employment Related   If the Employment Related box is checked, it means that the illness or accident is in some way related to a patient's employment.

Emergency   If a patient sees the provider on an emergency visit, a check mark is entered in the Emergency box.

Accident—Related To The Accident—Related To box indicates whether a patient's condition is related to an accident. The drop-down list offers three choices: Auto, if it is related to an automobile accident; No, if it is not accident-related; and Yes, if it is accident-related but not an auto accident. If a patient's condition is accident-related, the State and Nature Of boxes should also be completed.

Accident—State The abbreviation for the state in which the accident occurred is entered in this box.

Accident—Nature of This box provides additional information about the type of accident. The following choices can be selected from the drop-down list: Injured at home, Injured at school, Injured during recreation, Motorcycle injury, Work injury/Non-collision, and Work injury/Self employed.

Dates—Unable to Work If a patient is unable to work, the dates of the absence from work are listed in these boxes.

Dates—Total Disability If a patient is totally disabled, the dates of the total disability are entered in these boxes.

Dates—Partial Disability If a patient is partially disabled, the dates of the partial disability are listed in these boxes.

Dates—Hospitalization If a patient is hospitalized, the dates of the hospitalization are entered in these boxes.

Last X-Ray Date The Last X-Ray Date box is used by chiropractic offices to list the date of a patient's last X ray.

Death Status The Death Status box indicates a patient's condition according to the Karnofsky Performance Status Scale. There are 11 options: Able to carry on normal activity, Cares for self, Dead, Disabled, Moribund (a terminal condition near death), Normal, Normal activity with effort, Requires considerable assistance, Requires occasional assistance, Severely disabled, and Very sick. If this information is not provided by the physician, the box should be left blank.

Workers' Compensation—Return to Work Indicator If a patient has been out of work on Workers' Compensation, the patient's return to work status is selected from the drop-down list of choices: Conditional, Limited, or Normal. If the status is Conditional or Limited, the Percent of Disability box should also be completed.

Workers' Compensation—Percent of Disability This box indicates a patient's percent of disability upon returning to work.

Exercise 6-5

Complete the Condition tab for Hiro Tanaka. The information needed to complete this exercise is found on Source Documents 1 and 3.

MediSoft Program Date: August 9, 2003

Windows System Date: August 9, 2003

1. Edit the case for Hiro Tanaka.

2. Make the Condition tab active.

3. Enter the date of the injury in the Injury/Illness/LMP Date box.

4. Leave the Illness Indicator box blank.

5. In the First Consultation Date box, enter the date Tanaka first saw Dr. Yan for this condition.

6. Since this visit resulted from a non work-related accident, leave the Date Similar Symptoms box, the Same/Similar Symptoms box, and the Employment Related box blank.

7. Since this was an emergency visit, place a check mark in the Emergency box by clicking it.

8. Complete the Accident—Related To box.

9. In the Accident—State box, enter the two-letter abbreviation for the state in which the accident occurred.

10. Tanaka was injured while driving home from a softball game. Complete the Accident—Nature Of box regarding the type of accident.

11. Enter the dates Tanaka was unable to work in the Dates—Unable to Work boxes.

12. Enter the dates Tanaka was totally disabled in the Dates—Total Disability boxes.

13. Enter the dates Tanaka was partially disabled in the Dates—Partial Disability boxes.

14. Enter the dates Tanaka was hospitalized in the Dates—Hospitalization boxes.

15. Leave the Last X-Ray Date box blank.

16. Complete the Death Status box.

17. Since Tanaka was not injured at work, the Workers' Compensation boxes should be left blank.

18. Check your work for accuracy.

19. Save the changes.

20. Do not close the Patient List dialog box.

MEDICAID AND CHAMPUS TAB

For patients covered by Medicaid or CHAMPUS, the Medicaid and CHAMPUS tab is used to enter additional information about the government program (see Figure 6-19).

Medicaid

EPSDT EPSDT stands for "Early and Periodic Screening, Diagnosis, and Treatment." This is a Medicaid program for patients under the age of 21 who need screening and diagnostic services to determine physical or mental problems as well as treatment for conditions discovered. It also includes well-baby checkup examinations. A check mark in the EPSDT box indicates that a patient's visit is part of the EPSDT program.

Family Planning A check mark in the Family Planning box specifies that a patient's condition is related to family planning.

Resubmission Number For claims being resubmitted to Medicaid, the resubmission number is entered in this box.

Original Reference For claims being resubmitted to Medicaid, the original reference number is recorded in the Original Reference box.

CHAMPUS

CHAMPUS is the Civilian Health and Medical Program of the Uniformed Services (Army, Navy, Air Force, Marine Corps, Coast Guard, Public Health Service, and the National Oceanic and Atmospheric

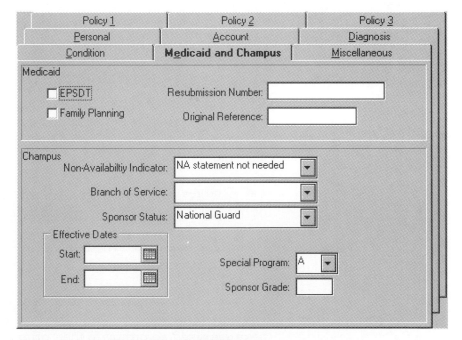

Figure 6-19 Medicaid and CHAMPUS tab.

Administration) that serves spouses and children of active-duty service members, military retirees and their families, some former spouses, and survivors of deceased military members.

Non-Availability Indicator The Non-Availability Indicator box specifies whether a nonavailability statement is required. The choices on the drop-down list are NA statement not needed, NA statement obtained, and Other carrier paid at least 75%.

Branch of Service The Branch of Service box indicates the particular branch of service: Air Force, Army, Champ VA, Coast Guard, Marines, Navy, NOAA, and Public Health Service.

sponsor an active-duty service member.

Sponsor Status The **sponsor** is the active-duty service member. The sponsor's family members are covered by the CHAMPUS insurance plan. The drop-down list in the Sponsor Status box provides choices to indicate the sponsor's status in the service, such as Active, Medal of Honor, Reserves, and so on.

Effective Dates The start date of the CHAMPUS policy is entered in the Effective Dates—Start box. If there is an end date, it is entered in the Effective Dates—End box. Specific dates can be entered, or a selection can be made from the pop-up calendar.

Special Program The Special Program drop-down list contains codes for special CHAMPUS programs.

Sponsor Grade The two-character sponsor grade is entered in the Sponsor Grade box.

MISCELLANEOUS TAB

The Miscellaneous tab records a variety of miscellaneous information about the patient and his or her treatment (see Figure 6-20).

Outside Lab Work If the Outside Lab Work box is checked, the lab work was performed by a lab other than the physician's office. If the lab bills the provider rather than the patient, then the provider bills the patient for the lab work even though it was performed by an outside lab.

Lab Charges The charges for lab work, whether performed inside or outside the practice, are entered in the Lab Charges box.

Local Use A and B These boxes may be used by some medical practices to record information specific to the local office.

Indicator If an indicator code is used to categorize patients or services, it is entered in the Indicator box. For example, patients might be categorized according to their primary diagnosis. Services might

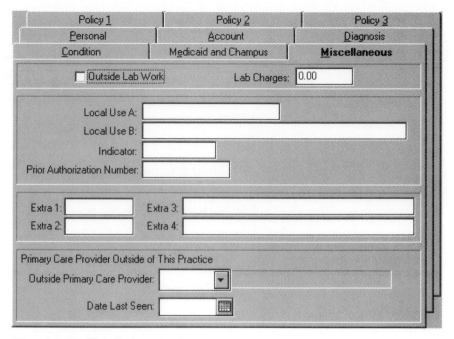

Figure 6-20 Miscellaneous tab.

be divided into such categories as lab work, consultations, hospital visits, and so on.

Prior Authorization Number   Before some services are performed, prior authorization must be obtained from the appropriate insurance carrier. If an insurance carrier has issued an authorization number for treatment that has not yet occurred, the number is entered in the Prior Authorization Number box.

Extra 1, 2, 3, and 4   The Extra 1, 2, 3, and 4 boxes are used for different purposes depending on the medical practice.

Outside Primary Care Provider   If a patient is covered by a managed care plan and the patient's primary care provider is outside the medical practice, the name of the provider is selected from the drop-down list in the Outside Primary Care Provider box.

Date Last Seen   The Date Last Seen box lists the date a patient was last seen by the outside primary care provider.

EDITING CASE INFORMATION ON AN ESTABLISHED PATIENT

Information in an existing case is modified by selecting the case to be edited and clicking the Edit Case button at the bottom of the Patient List dialog box. (The Case radio button must be clicked for the Edit Case button to be displayed.)

Exercise 6-6

John Fitzwilliams, an established patient, has just remarried. Edit the information in his Case dialog box to reflect this change.

MediSoft Program Date: March 10, 2003

Windows System Date: March 10, 2003

1. Edit the case for John Fitzwilliams.

2. In the Personal tab, change the entry in the Marital Status box from Divorced to Married.

3. Check your work for accuracy.

4. Save the changes.

5. Close the Patient List dialog box.

6. Exit MediSoft.

CHAPTER REVIEW

USING TERMINOLOGY

Match the terms on the left with the definitions on the right.

_____ **1.** capitated plan

_____ **2.** cases

_____ **3.** chart

_____ **4.** Medigap

_____ **5.** record of treatment and progress

_____ **6.** referring provider

_____ **7.** sponsor

a. A folder that contains a patient's medical records.

b. Physician's notes about a patient's condition and diagnosis.

c. A physician who recommends that a patient make an appointment with another specific physician.

d. A private insurance plan that supplements Medicare coverage.

e. An insurance plan in which payments are made to primary care providers for patients whether they have an office visit or not.

f. Groupings of transactions organized around a patient's condition.

g. The active-duty service member on the CHAMPUS government program.

CHECKING YOUR UNDERSTANDING

Answer the questions below in the space provided.

8. Sarina Bell has no insurance of her own but is covered by her father's insurance policy. How would this be indicated in the Policy 1 tab for Sarina Bell?

_____

_____

9. Where in the Case dialog box can you find information about a patient's allergies?

_____

_____

10. Is it necessary to set up a new case when a patient changes insurance carriers? Why or why not?

_____

_____

11. In the Case dialog box, where would you enter information about a work-related accident?

_____

_____

12. Where is information needed to complete the Diagnosis tab usually found?

_____

_____

13. A patient has been seeing the doctor regularly for treatment of diabetes. Yesterday she was hospitalized, and the doctor saw her in the hospital for treatment. Do you need to set up a new case for the hospitalization?

_____

_____

APPLYING KNOWLEDGE

Answer the questions below in the space provided.

14. While you are entering case information for a new patient, you realize that the patient's referring provider is not one of the choices in the Referring Provider box in the Account tab. What should you do?

_____

_____

15. One of the established patients has changed insurance carriers from Blue Cross/Blue Shield to OhioCare HMO. What specific boxes need to be changed in the Case dialog box?

_____

_____

AT THE COMPUTER

Answer the following question at the computer:

16. Using Source Documents 2 and 5, create a new case for patient Juanita Ramos. Fill in the Personal, Account, Diagnosis, and Policy 1 tabs.

7 Entering Transactions

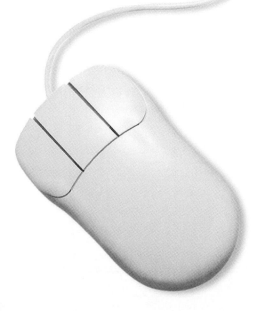

WHAT YOU NEED TO KNOW

To use this chapter, you need to know how to:

◆ Start MediSoft, use menus, and enter and edit text.

◆ Edit information in an existing case.

◆ Work with chart and case numbers.

OBJECTIVES

In this chapter, you will learn how to:

◆ Record information about patients' visits, including procedure codes and charges.

◆ Record payments received from patients and insurers.

◆ Enter adjustments to charges.

◆ Edit transactions.

◆ Use MediSoft's Briefcase button and Locate feature to find specific transaction data.

◆ Print walkout receipts.

KEY TERMS

adjustments
charges
modifiers

MultiLink codes
payments

TRANSACTION ENTRY OVERVIEW

charges *the amounts a provider bills for services performed.*

payments *monies received from patients and insurance carriers.*

adjustments *changes to patients' accounts.*

Three types of transactions are recorded in MediSoft: charges, payments, and adjustments. **Charges** are the amounts a provider bills for the services performed. **Payments** are monies received from patients and insurance carriers. **Adjustments** are changes to patients' accounts. Examples of adjustments include returned check fees, insurance write-offs, Medicare adjustments, changes in treatment, and so on.

The main document needed to enter billing transactions in MediSoft is a patient's superbill (also called a charge ticket or encounter form). Charges and payments listed on a superbill are entered in the Transaction Entry dialog box in MediSoft. After the information is entered, it is checked for accuracy. If all the information is correct, the transaction data is saved and a walkout receipt is printed for the patient. If it is incorrect, the data is edited and then saved.

THE TRANSACTION ENTRY DIALOG BOX

Transactions are entered in the Transaction Entry dialog box, which is accessed by clicking Enter Transactions on the Activities menu (see Figure 7-1). The Transaction Entry dialog box lists existing transactions and provides options for creating new transactions and for editing existing transactions. All transactions entered in Medi-Soft begin with two critical pieces of information: a patient's chart number and the case number, which is related to the procedures per-

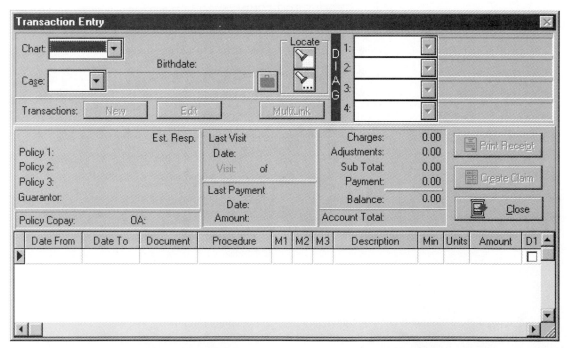

Figure 7-1 Transaction Entry dialog box.

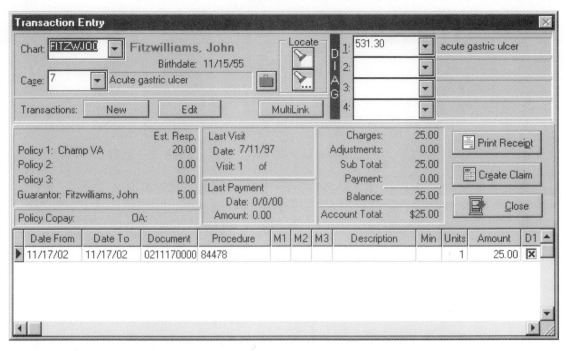

Figure 7-2 Transaction Entry dialog box with case data displayed.

formed. The chart number and case number must be selected in the Transaction Entry dialog box before a transaction can be entered. Boxes for entering these are found at the top left of the dialog box.

Chart   To begin entering a new transaction, a patient's chart number is clicked on the drop-down list in the Chart box. Many practices have long lists of chart numbers in MediSoft. The fastest way to enter a chart number is to key the first few letters of the patient's last name, which then displays that location in the drop-down list of chart numbers.

Case   After the chart number has been selected, the Case box displays a case number and description for a particular patient (see Figure 7-2). If a patient has more than one open case, the drop-down list displays the full list of cases.

After the chart and case numbers have been entered, a new transaction can be created or an existing transaction can be edited. Transactions already in the system for a patient whose chart number is active are listed at the bottom of the dialog box. The scroll bar at the bottom of the dialog box may be used to display a full summary of the transaction (see Figure 7-3 on page 120).

The process of creating a new transaction in MediSoft begins with clicking the New button. When the New button is clicked, three transaction entry tabs appear: Charge, Payment, and Adjustment, as described in the following sections of this chapter.

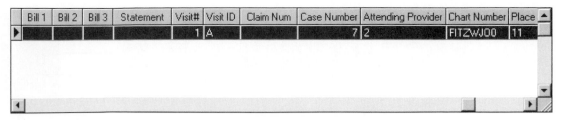

Figure 7-3 *Information displayed when scrolling to the right.*

ENTERING CHARGES

Charges for procedures are entered in the Charge tab (see Figure 7-4). This tab contains the following boxes:

Dates In the Dates boxes, the system automatically defaults to the current date, that is, the MediSoft Program Date. If this is not the date that the procedures were performed, the data in the Dates boxes need to be changed to reflect the actual date of the procedures. Data in these boxes can be changed by keying over the information that is already there. New dates can also be selected by clicking the Pop-up Calendar buttons beside the Dates boxes.

To change the default date for these boxes, either of these methods is used:

◆ The Set Program Date command on the File menu is clicked, or

◆ The Date button in the bottom-right corner of the screen is clicked. (This must be done before the New button is clicked in the Transaction Entry dialog box.)

Document The system displays a document number automatically; it is the current date (listed in YYMMDD format instead of the usual MMDDYY format) followed by four zeros. Medical offices use different systems for creating document numbers. Some offices use a system in which every superbill number starts with the date and is followed by a different number for each patient seen that day. Other offices use the superbill number as the document number. Up to 10 characters can be entered. For the purposes of this text/workbook, use the default document numbers assigned by the system.

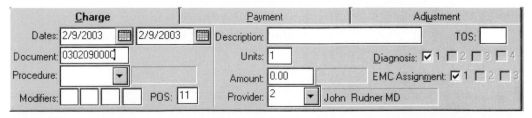

Figure 7-4 Charge tab.

Procedure   The procedure code for a service performed is selected from the drop-down list of CPT codes already entered in the system. Only one procedure code can be selected for each transaction. If multiple procedures were performed for a patient, each one must be entered as a separate transaction (unless a MultiLink code, which is discussed in the next paragraph, is being used). After the CPT code is selected from the drop-down list and the Tab key or Enter key is pressed, the charge for a procedure is displayed in the Amount box. If the CPT code is not listed, it will need to be added to the database by clicking Procedure/Payment/Adjustment Codes on the Lists menu. This may be done without exiting the Transaction Entry dialog box.

MULTILINK CODES

MultiLink codes groups of procedure code entries that relate to a single activity.

MediSoft provides a feature that saves time when entering multiple CPT codes that are related. **MultiLink codes** are groups of procedure code entries that relate to a single activity. Using MultiLink codes saves time by eliminating the need to enter related multiple procedure codes one at a time. For example, suppose a MultiLink code is created for the procedures related to diagnosing a strep throat. The MultiLink code STREPM is created. STREPM includes three procedures: 99211 Minimal Visit, 87072 Strep Culture, and 85022 CBC w/Diff.

When the MultiLink code STREPM is selected, all three procedure codes are entered automatically by the system, eliminating the need to make three different entries. The MultiLink feature saves time by reducing the number of procedure code entries, and it also reduces omission errors. If procedure codes are entered in a MultiLink, it is impossible to forget to enter a procedure, since all of the codes that are in the MultiLink group are entered automatically.

MultiLink

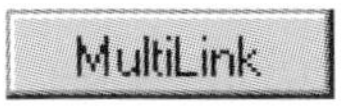

Figure 7-5 MultiLink button.

Clicking the MultiLink button (see Figure 7-5) in the Transaction Entry dialog box displays the MultiLink dialog box. After a MultiLink code is selected from the MultiLink drop-down list, the Create Transactions button is clicked. The codes and charges for each procedure are automatically added to the list of transactions at the bottom of the Transaction Entry dialog box.

modifiers one- or two-digit codes that allow a more specific description to be entered for services performed.

Modifiers   Some CPT codes have modifiers. **Modifiers** are one- or two-digit codes that allow a more specific description to be entered for the services the physician performed. For example, a modifier needs to be used when the circumstances require services beyond those normally associated with a particular procedure code. If a modifier is indicated on a superbill, it is entered in the Modifiers box. There can be up to four modifiers for each procedure code.

POS   The POS, or Place of Service box, indicates where services were performed. The standard numerical codes used are:

11	Provider's office
21	Inpatient hospital
22	Outpatient hospital
23	Hospital emergency room

When MediSoft is set up for use in a practice, an option is provided to set a default POS code. For purposes of this text/workbook, the default code has been set to 11 for Provider's office.

Description   The Description box is normally left blank in the Charge tab.

Units   The Units box indicates the quantity of the procedure. Normally, the number of units is one. In some cases, however, it may be more than one. For example, if a patient was seen by a physician for three days of hospital visits and the charge linked to the CPT code is for one day, "3" would be entered in the Units box.

Amount   The Amount box lists the charge amount for a procedure performed. The amount is entered automatically by the system based on the CPT code. Each CPT code stored in the system has a charge amount associated with it. The charge amount can be edited if necessary. To the right of the Amount box is the Extended Amount area. This area displays the total charges for the procedure(s) performed. The amount is calculated by the system; the number in the Units box is multiplied by the number in the Amount box. For example, suppose a patient had three X rays done at a charge of $45.00 per X ray. The Units box would read "3," and the Amount box would read "$45.00." The Extended Amount box would read "$135.00," which is 3 x $45.00.

Provider   The Provider box lists the code number and name of a patient's assigned provider. If a patient sees a different provider for a visit, the Provider box can be changed to list that provider instead.

TOS   TOS stands for "type of service." Medical offices may set up a list of codes to indicate the type of service performed. For example, 1 may indicate an examination, 2 a lab test, and so on.

Diagnosis   The Diagnosis 1, 2, 3, and 4 check boxes in the Charge tab correspond to the DIAG 1, 2, 3, and 4 boxes in the main Transaction Entry dialog box. A check mark appears in each Diagnosis box for which a diagnosis was entered in the DIAG 1, 2, 3, 4 boxes. Check marks can be deleted if appropriate.

EMC Assignment   The 1, 2, and 3 boxes represent up to three insurance policies for transmitting electronic media claims. The 1, 2, and 3 boxes correspond to the insurance carriers listed in the Policy 1, Policy 2, and Policy 3 tabs in a patient's Case dialog box.

SAVING CHARGE TRANSACTIONS

When all the charge information has been entered and checked for accuracy, it needs to be saved. When a transaction is saved, it is added to the list at the bottom of the Transaction Entry dialog box, along with other transactions that have already been entered for the case.

Transactions are saved in MediSoft by clicking one of the buttons grouped vertically at the right side of the Transaction Entry dialog box:

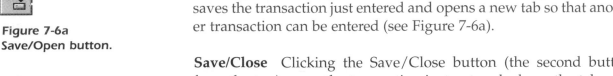

Figure 7-6a
Save/Open button.

Save/Open   Clicking the Save/Open button at the top of the group saves the transaction just entered and opens a new tab so that another transaction can be entered (see Figure 7-6a).

Figure 7-6b
Save/Close button.

Save/Close   Clicking the Save/Close button (the second button from the top) saves the transaction just entered, closes the tab, and redisplays the main Transaction Entry dialog box (see Figure 7-6b).

Figure 7-6c
Cancel button.

Cancel   The Cancel button displays a red "X." This button deletes the transaction data just entered and redisplays the main Transaction Entry dialog box (see Figure 7-6c).

Figure 7-6d
Transaction Documentation button.

Transaction Documentation   When the Transaction Documentation button (located at the bottom of the group) (see Figure 7-6d) is clicked, the Transaction Documentation dialog box is displayed (see Figure 7-7). This dialog box is used to provide additional information about a particular transaction. The Transaction Documentation dialog box is optional; it only has to be completed when there is additional information about a particular transaction that needs to be recorded. MediSoft provides several types of transaction documentation. For example, in the Type drop-down list, a variety of choices are listed, such as Diagnostic Report, Operative Note, and Transaction Note (internal use only). After information is entered in the Documentation/Notes box, it is saved by clicking the OK

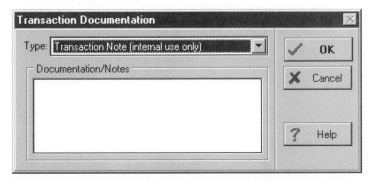

Figure 7-7 Transaction Documentation dialog box.

button. The information can be deleted by clicking the Cancel button. A Help button is also available within the Transaction Documentation dialog box.

Exercise 7-1

Using Source Document 6, complete the Charge tab for Elizabeth Jones' diabetes case.

MediSoft Program Date: December 8, 2003

1. Start MediSoft and change the MediSoft Program Date.

2. On the Activities menu, click Enter Transactions. The Transaction Entry dialog box is displayed.

3. Key *JONES* in the Chart box to select Elizabeth Jones. Verify that the Diabetes case is the active case in the Case box.

4. Click the New button. The Charge tab is displayed.

5. Accept the default in the Dates boxes (12/08/03).

6. Accept the default entry in the Document box (0312080000).

7. Key *99213* in the Procedure box to select the procedure code for the services checked off on the superbill.

8. Since there are no modifiers to the procedure code, the Modifiers boxes are left blank.

9. Accept the default entry of 11 in the POS box.

10. Leave the Description box blank.

11. Keep "1" in the Units box.

12. Accept the charge for the procedure that is displayed in the Amount box ($100.00).

13. Accept the information displayed in the Provider box, leave the TOS box blank, and accept the information in the Diagnosis and EMC Assignment boxes.

14. Check your entries for accuracy.

15. Click the Save/Close button to return to the main Transaction Entry dialog box. This is accomplished by clicking the second button from the top in the group of buttons at the right side of the dialog box. Notice that the transaction just entered is now listed at the bottom of the dialog box.

Exercise 7-2

Using Source Document 7, complete the Charge tab for John Fitzwilliams' acute gastric ulcer case.

MediSoft Program Date: December 8, 2003

1. If necessary, open the Transaction Entry dialog box.

2. In the Chart box, key *FITZ*. Notice that the chart number for John Fitzwilliams is highlighted on the drop-down list. Press the Tab key. Verify that "Acute gastric ulcer" is the active case in the Case box.

3. Click the New button. The Charge tab becomes active.

4. Accept the default in the Dates boxes (12/08/03).

5. Accept the default entry in the Document box (0312080000).

6. Select the procedure code for the services checked off on the superbill. Notice there is more than one procedure. Select the first procedure code (80019).

7. Since there are no modifiers to the procedure code, the Modifiers boxes are left blank.

8. Accept the default entry of 11 in the POS box.

9. Leave the Description box blank.

10. Keep "1" in the Units box.

11. Accept the charge for the procedure that is displayed in the Amount box ($80.00).

12. Accept the information displayed in the Provider box, leave the TOS box blank, and accept the information displayed in the Diagnosis and EMC Assignment boxes.

13. Check your entries for accuracy.

14. Click the Save/Open button. This is the first of four buttons grouped on the right side of the dialog box.

15. Accept the default in the Dates boxes.

16. Accept the default entry in the Document box.

17. Select the procedure code for the second service checked off on the superbill (84478).

18. Since there are no modifiers to the procedure code, the Modifiers boxes are left blank.

19. Accept the default entry in the POS box.

20. Leave the Description box blank.

21. Keep "1" in the Units box.

22. Accept the charge for the procedure that is displayed in the Amount box ($25.00).

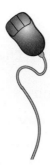

23. Accept the information displayed in the Provider box, leave the TOS box blank, and accept the information displayed in the Diagnosis and EMC Assignment boxes.

24. Check your entries for accuracy.

25. Click the Save/Close button to return to the main Transaction Entry dialog box. Notice that the two transactions just entered are now listed at the bottom of the dialog box.

26. Close the Transaction Entry dialog box.

ENTERING PAYMENTS

Payments from patients and insurance carriers are entered in the Payment tab of the Transaction Entry dialog box (see Figure 7-8). Before entering a payment, it is important to look at the list of charges displayed at the bottom of the Transaction Entry dialog box. The document number for a charge being paid must be identified. When information is entered about a payment, the document number that corresponds to the charge must be used so that the payment is applied to the correct charge. The Payment tab contains the following boxes:

Date   In the Date box, the date when the payment was received is entered. The value in this box defaults to the current date (MediSoft Program Date).

Document   The Document box must display the document number of the transaction to which the payment is being applied. The default entry in this box uses the current date, not the date of the original charge. *It is important that the payment document number matches the document number of the original transaction, so the system knows which charge is being paid. Thus, in most cases the default entry in the Document box must be changed.*

Pay Code   From the drop-down list in the Pay Code box, the type of payment is selected. For purposes of this text/workbook, the codes are:

01   Patient payment, cash

02   Patient payment, check

03   Insurance carrier payment

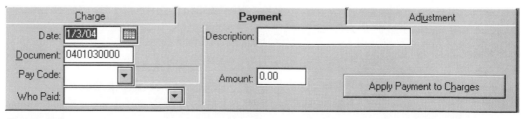

Figure 7-8 Payment tab.

Who Paid From the drop-down list in the Who Paid box, the party that made the payment is selected. The choices include the patient and the patient's insurance carrier(s).

Description If a payment is made by check, the check number is entered in the Description box. If a payment is not made by check, the Description box can be used to record other information about the payment.

Amount The amount of a payment is entered in the Amount box.

APPLYING PAYMENTS TO CHARGES

After the Payment tab's boxes have been completed and checked for accuracy, the payment must be applied to charges. This is accomplished by clicking the Apply Payment to Charges button. The Apply Payment to Charges dialog box is then displayed (see Figure 7-9). The dialog box lists information about all unpaid charges for a patient, including the date of the procedure, the document number, the procedure code, the charge, the balance, and the total amount paid. In the top right corner of the dialog box, the amount of payment that has not yet been applied to charges is listed in the Unapplied box. The cursor appears in the first box of the column labeled "This Payment." Clicking on the zeros in the This Payment box moves the zeros to the top left corner of the box. This indicates that the box is active and ready for entry. The amount of a payment that is to be applied to a charge is entered without a decimal point.

Payments can be applied to more than one charge. For example, suppose that the amount in the Unapplied box is $200 and there are three charges that have not been paid. The $200 payment can be

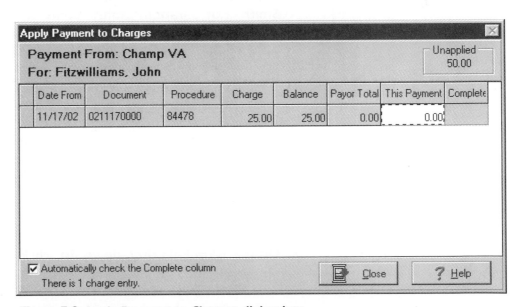

Figure 7-9 Apply Payment to Charges dialog box.

applied to one of the charges or two of the charges, or it can be distributed among the three charges. It is not even necessary to apply the entire payment amount. A balance can remain in the Unapplied box, or the balance can be used to reduce the amount due on another charge.

Clicking the Close button exits the Apply Payment to Charges dialog box and the Payment tab is again displayed. In the list of transactions at the bottom of the Transaction Entry dialog box, the payment is now listed.

SAVING PAYMENT TRANSACTIONS

When all the information on a payment has been entered and checked for accuracy, it must be saved. Payment transactions are saved in the manner described earlier for charge transactions. The Transaction Documentation feature is also available in the Payment tab.

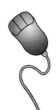

Exercise 7-3

Sarabeth Smith is a managed care patient. Every time she sees her primary care physician, Dr. Jessica Rudner, she pays a $15 co-payment. Even though no insurance claim will be filed, Ms. Smith's payment must be recorded in MediSoft. Enter a payment of $15 received from Sarabeth Smith for services provided on April 23, 2003. Her check number is 1017.

MediSoft Program Date: April 23, 2003

1. Open the Transaction Entry dialog box.

2. In the Chart box, key SMITHS and press Tab to select Sarabeth Smith. Notice that "SMITHS" was keyed instead of "SMITH," because "SMITH" displayed the chart number of James L. Smith, not Sarabeth Smith. Verify that "Chest pain" is the active case in the Case box.

3. Click the New button. Make the Payment tab active.

4. Accept the default entry of 4/23/03 in the Date box.

5. The entry in the Document box must match the document number for the charge entry to which this payment should be applied. Look at the document number for the charge entry (listed in the bottom section of the dialog box), and verify that the document number in the Payment tab matches the entry for the charge.

6. On the Pay Code drop-down list, click 02, patient payment, check.

7. On the Who Paid drop-down list, click Smith, Sarabeth.

8. Enter the check number in the Description box.

9. Enter the amount of the payment in the Amount box. Press the Tab key.

10. Click the Apply Payment to Charges button. The Apply Payment to Charges dialog box is displayed.

11. Notice that the amount of this payment ($15.00) is listed in the Unapplied box at the top right of the dialog box.

12. Click the zeros in the This Payment box. Notice that they move to the top left of the box.

13. Key *15* in the This Payment box. Press the Tab key. Notice that the system inserts a decimal point.

14. Click the Close button. The Payment tab is displayed again.

15. Click the Save/Close button to return to the main Transaction Entry dialog box.

16. Check your entries for accuracy. Notice that the payment just entered is now listed at the bottom of the dialog box and that the amount displayed in the Account Total box in the middle of the dialog box is now zero.

17. Close the Transaction Entry dialog box.

Exercise 7-4

Enter a payment of $84 received from John Fitzwilliams's insurance carrier for services provided on December 8, 2003. The insurance carrier is paying 80 percent ($84) of the total charges for that day ($105). The check number is 214778924.

MediSoft Program Date: December 8, 2003

1. Open the Transaction Entry dialog box.

2. In the Chart box, key *FITZ* to select John Fitzwilliams. Verify that the Acute gastric ulcer case is displayed in the Case box.

3. Click the New button. Click the Payment tab to make it active.

4. Accept the default entry of 12/08/03 in the Date box.

5. Verify that the entry in the Document box matches the document number entered for the charge transaction to which the payment should be applied. Notice that there are two charges for this date with the same document number. Payments must be applied to the charges one at a time.

6. On the Pay Code drop-down list, click 03, insurance carrier payment.

7. On the Who Paid drop-down list, click Champ VA.

8. Enter the check number in the Description box.

9. In the Amount box, enter the amount of the payment. Press the Tab key.

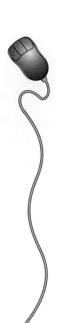

10. Click the Apply Payment to Charges button.

11. In the This Payment box, click the first charge entry that has a document number that matches the document number for the payment (0312080000).

12. Key *80* in the This Payment box, because 80 is the total amount of the charge for this procedure. Press the Enter key. Notice that $4.00 is now listed in the Unapplied box.

13. In the This Payment box, click the second charge entry for December 8, 2003.

14. Key *4* in the This Payment box. Press the Enter key. Notice that the amount in the Unapplied box is now down to zero.

15. Click the Close button. The Payment tab is displayed again.

16. Click the Save/Close button.

17. Check your entries for accuracy. Notice that the payment just entered is now listed at the bottom of the dialog box.

18. Close the Transaction Entry dialog box.

ENTERING ADJUSTMENTS

Sometimes a change, or an adjustment, needs to be made to a patient's account. For example, a patient laid off from work may speak with his or her physician about the possibility of reducing a bill. The amount of the reduction needs to be entered in MediSoft. Many times insurance carriers do not pay claims in full. Payment may be 80 percent or 50 percent of the charges, or some other percent. This information is found on the explanation of benefits (EOB) that accompanies payments. Sometimes an EOB includes an explanation of what is being paid or not being paid and why. When a medical office receives an EOB, an adjustment transaction may need to be entered.

The Adjustment tab is used for making changes or corrections in a patient's account (see Figure 7-10). This tab contains the following boxes:

Date The date of the original transaction is entered in the Date box.

Document The document number of an original charge is entered in the Document box.

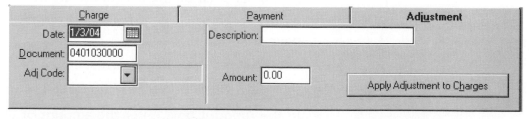

Figure 7-10 Adjustment tab.

Adj Code   The type of adjustment is selected from the list of choices in the Adj Code drop-down list. Examples of types of adjustments include Insurance company adjustments, Patient adjustments, and so on.

Description   Information that describes an adjustment is entered in the Description box.

Amount   The amount of an adjustment is entered in the Amount box. If an adjustment reduces the amount owed, a minus sign must be entered in front of the numerals.

APPLYING ADJUSTMENTS TO CHARGES   When the Adjustment tab's boxes have been completed and checked for accuracy, the Apply Adjustment to Charges button is clicked. The Apply Adjustment to Charges dialog box is displayed (see Figure 7-11). All charges for a patient are listed in the dialog box. The amount of an adjustment is listed in the Unapplied box at the top right corner of the dialog box. The cursor is in the first box in the This Adjust column. Clicking the zeros in the This Adjust box moves the zeros to the top left corner of the box. This indicates that the box is active and ready for entry. The dollar amount of an adjustment is entered with a minus sign before the number if the adjustment will reduce a patient's balance. The adjustment is then applied to the charge that it is adjusting. When the total adjustment is applied, the amount listed in the Unapplied box is zero. Clicking the Close button exits the Apply Adjustment to Charges dialog box, and the Adjustment tab is displayed. In the list of transactions at the bottom of the Transaction Entry dialog box, the adjustment is now listed.

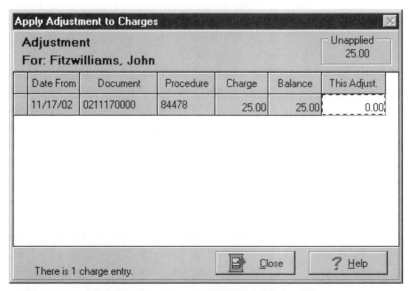

Figure 7-11 Apply Adjustment to Charges dialog box.

SAVING ADJUSTMENT TRANSACTIONS

When all the information on an adjustment has been entered and checked for accuracy, it must be saved. Adjustment transactions are saved in the manner described earlier for charge and payment transactions. The Transaction Documentation feature is also available in the Adjustment tab.

Exercise 7-5

The medical office has received an EOB from East Ohio PPO for Sarina Bell. The original charge for the procedure was $100, but East Ohio PPO is paying $70 instead of $80. Enter a payment of $70.00 and an adjustment of -$10. The check number is 9042739.

MediSoft Program Date: December 22, 2003

1. Open the Transaction Entry dialog box.

2. In the Chart box, key *BELLSAR* to select Sarina Bell. Verify that the Ear ache case is displayed in the Case box.

3. Click the New button. Click the Payment tab to make it active.

4. Accept the default entry in the Date box. This date reflects the date the payment was received.

5. In the Document box, enter the document number of the charge for which this insurance payment has been received. This document number is listed in the bottom half of the dialog box, in the column titled "Document." In this exercise, it is 0306100000.

6. On the Pay Code drop-down list, click 03, insurance carrier payment.

7. On the Who Paid drop-down list, click East Ohio PPO.

8. Enter the check number in the Description box.

9. Key *70* in the Amount box. Press the Tab key.

10. Click the Apply Payment to Charges button. Notice that the amount of this payment ($70.00) is listed in the Unapplied box at the top right of the dialog box.

11. Click the zeros in the This Payment box. Notice that they move to the top left of the box.

12. Key *70* in the This Payment box. Press the Enter key.

13. Click the Close button. The Payment tab is displayed again.

14. Click the Save/Open button.

15. Click the Adjustment tab to make it active.

16. Accept the default entry in the Date box, since this is the date the adjustment is being made.

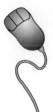

17. In the Document box, enter the document number for the charge to which the adjustment is being applied (0306100000).

18. On the Adj Code drop-down list, click 04, insurance company adjustment.

19. In the Description box, enter East Ohio PPO Adj.

20. Key *-10* in the Amount box. Press the Tab key.

21. Click the Apply Adjustment to Charges button. Notice that the amount of this adjustment (-10.00) is listed in the Unapplied box at the top right of the dialog box.

22. Click in the This Adjustment box. Notice that the zeros move to the top left of the box.

23. Key *-10* in the This Adjustment box, without a decimal point. Press the Tab key.

24. Click the Close button.

25. Click the Save/Close button.

26. Check your entries for accuracy. Notice that the payment and adjustment just entered are now listed at the bottom of the Transaction Entry dialog box. Also notice that the amount in the Account Total box is now $20.00, the amount still owed by the patient.

27. Close the Transaction Entry dialog box.

PRINTING WALKOUT RECEIPTS

After transactions have been entered in the Transaction Entry dialog box, a walkout receipt can be printed for a patient. Walkout receipts are usually printed when a patient makes a payment before leaving the office. In these instances, walkout receipts are printed from within the Transaction Entry dialog box. If desired, a walkout receipt can be printed at a later time via the Custom Report List option on the Reports menu.

A walkout receipt includes information on the procedures, diagnosis, and charges for a visit. A patient can attach the receipt to an insurance form and submit it directly to his or her carrier. If there is a balance due, the receipt serves as a reminder to the patient of the amount owed. In the Transaction Entry dialog box, a walkout receipt is printed by clicking the Print Receipt button. The Open Report dialog box is displayed, and the available reports are listed under the Report Title heading (see Figure 7-12). Click Walkout Receipt to select the report title, and then click the OK button. MediSoft then asks whether the report is to be previewed on the screen or sent directly to the printer. If the report is to be previewed on screen, it

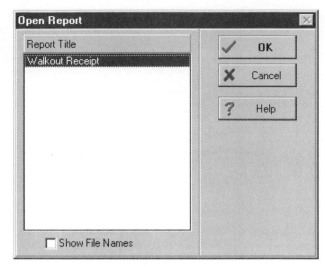

Figure 7-12 Open Report dialog box.

can subsequently be printed directly from the Preview Report window. After the preview/print choice has been made, the Data Selection Questions dialog box is displayed that confirms the patient's chart number and case number, as well as the date of the transaction. The system automatically enters default data in these boxes based upon the transaction that is active. Clicking the OK button accepts the default data and sends the report to the printer.

When a walkout receipt is printed, it lists the current date (the actual date the receipt is printed) at the top. MediSoft uses the Windows System Date for this information, not the MediSoft Program Date. If the Windows date differs from the program date set in MediSoft, the date at the top of the walkout receipt will not agree with the date of the transaction in MediSoft. These two dates should be the same.

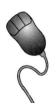

Exercise 7-6

Enter a cash payment of $8 for Samuel Bell's office visit on February 3, 2003. Since Samuel's insurance covers 80 percent of the charges, Samuel's father, Herbert, who is the guarantor, owes $8. Record the payment, and print a walkout receipt for the patient.

MediSoft Program Date: February 3, 2003

Windows System Date: February 3, 2003

1. Open the Transaction Entry dialog box.

2. In the Chart box, key *BELLS* to select Samuel Bell. Press the Tab key.

3. Verify that "Swollen neck glands" is displayed in the Case box.

4. Click the New button. Click the Payment tab to make it active.

5. Accept the default entry in the Date box, since this is the date the payment is received.

6. Verify that the entry in the Document box matches the document number for the charge transaction to which the payment is being applied.

7. On the Pay Code drop-down list, click 01, Patient payment, cash.

8. On the Who Paid drop-down list, click Bell, Samuel.

9. Leave the Description box blank.

10. In the Amount box, Key 8. Press the Tab key.

11. Click the Apply Payment to Charges button.

12. Click the This Payment box.

13. Key *8* in the This Payment box. Press the Tab key.

14. Click the Close button. The Payment tab is displayed again.

15. Click the Save/Close button.

16. Check your entries for accuracy.

17. Click the Print Receipt button. The Open Report dialog box is displayed.

18. Verify that Walkout Receipt is highlighted and then click the OK button.

19. In the Print Report Where? dialog box, click Print the report on the printer. Click the Start button.

20. The Print dialog box is displayed. Verify that the settings are correct and click the OK button.

21. The Data Selection Questions dialog box is displayed. Review the default entries and click the OK button to print the receipt.

22. Check the printed receipt for accuracy.

23. Close the Transaction Entry dialog box and reset the Windows System Date to the current date.

EDITING AND DELETING TRANSACTIONS

All transactions entered in MediSoft can be edited within the Transaction Entry dialog box. Double-clicking a particular transaction from the list at the bottom of the Transaction Entry dialog box is the fastest way to edit a transaction in MediSoft. Double-clicking opens the transaction and displays the original Charge, Payment, or Adjustment tab, where information can be changed. After changes are made, the data must be saved.

Transactions can also be deleted from the Transaction Entry dialog box. Clicking the transaction on the list at the bottom of the dialog box highlights the transaction. Once the transaction is highlighted, clicking the right-mouse button brings up a shortcut menu. The shortcut menu lists the following commands: Edit Transaction, New Transaction, and Delete Transaction. Clicking Delete Transaction causes a Confirm dialog box to be displayed, asking "Are you sure you want to delete this record?" Clicking the Yes button deletes the transaction; clicking the No button cancels the action.

LOCATING INFORMATION ON PATIENTS AND CASES

Sometimes it is necessary to locate certain patients or cases before editing. MediSoft provides two features within the Transaction Entry dialog box that make it easy to locate transaction information. The Briefcase button is used to find cases for a specific patient. The Locate feature provides powerful search capabilities for searching for a range of information.

Figure 7-13
Briefcase button.

Briefcase Button

The Briefcase button provides the opportunity to select cases for a particular patient by transaction date, procedure code, and/or amount (see Figure 7-13). This action is accomplished in the Select Case by Transaction Date dialog box (see Figure 7-14). The right side of this dialog box lists all transactions in the system for a particular patient. The left side contains several boxes that can be used to locate transactions that match certain criteria. These boxes are Date From, Procedure Code, and Amount. Any combination of the procedure dates, and/or transaction amounts can be entered in their respective boxes.

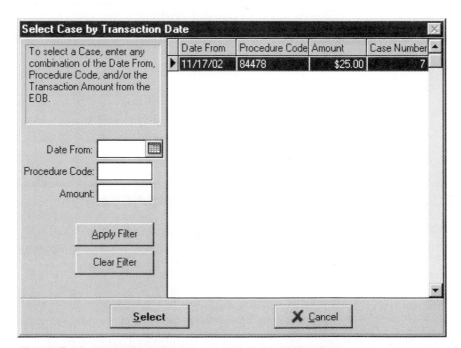

Figure 7-14 Select Case by Transaction Date dialog box.

For example, suppose a billing clerk needs to locate all transactions for procedures completed during an office visit on May 23, 2003. To search for that information, the patient's chart number would be selected in the Chart box, and then the Briefcase button would be clicked. In the Select Case by Transaction Date dialog box, "052303" would be entered in the Date From box and then the Apply Filter button would be clicked. Instead of listing all transactions for the patient, the right side of the dialog box now lists only those transactions performed on May 23, 2003. Similarly, a search can be conducted by procedure code or amount. Searches can be conducted using just one of the criteria, or they may include two or three criteria. When the Clear Filter button is clicked, the full list of transactions is displayed again on the right side of the dialog box. Clicking the Select button selects the particular transaction to which the arrow is pointing. The Cancel button closes the dialog box without making any selection.

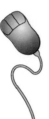

Exercise 7-7

Using the Briefcase button, locate all transactions for Randall Klein that contain Procedure Code 99212.

MediSoft Program Date: March 3, 2003

1. Open the Transaction Entry dialog box.

2. Key *KLE* in the Chart box to select Randall Klein. Press the Enter key.

3. Click the Briefcase button. The Select Case by Transaction Date dialog box is displayed. Notice that there are three transactions listed for Randall Klein.

4. In the Procedure Code box, key *99212*.

5. Click the Apply Filter button to begin the search. All transactions that do not match the search criteria are hidden from view; only the transaction that matches CPT code 99212 remains visible.

6. Click the Select button to select this transaction. The Transaction Entry dialog box is displayed again.

7. Close the Transaction Entry dialog box.

**Figure 7-15
Locate buttons.**

Locate Buttons

While the Briefcase button is used to search for cases of a particular patient, the Locate buttons (with flashlight icons) are used to perform searches for many types of information, including assigned provider, employer, date of birth, last payment amount, and so forth (see Figure 7-15).

When the top Locate button is clicked, the Locate Patient dialog box appears (see Figure 7-16). The bottom Locate button is used to find the next patient who matches the search criteria entered in the Locate Patient dialog box.

The Locate Patient dialog box contains the following boxes:

Field Value In the Field Value box, the specific characters that match or come close to matching the sought-after information are entered. For example, if someone were searching for a patient with the last name of Silverman, "Silverman" would be entered in the Field Value box. If a search were being conducted for patients of Dr. Singh, "Singh" would be entered.

Search Type The boxes in the Search Type area of the Locate Patient dialog box provide options that limit the parameters of the search.

> **Case Sensitive** A check mark in the Case Sensitive box indicates that the items found in the search must match the case of the characters entered in the Field Value box. If this box were checked, a search for "singh" would not return any matches, since the provider's name is in the database as "Singh," with an uppercase "S."

> **Exact Match** A check mark in the Exact Match box signifies that only information that exactly matches the entry in the Field Value box will be returned in the search.

> **Partial Match at Beginning** If the Partial Match at Beginning box is checked, the system will return items that match the beginning characters entered in the Field Value box.

> **Partial Match Anywhere** If the Partial Match Anywhere box is checked, the system will return items that match the characters

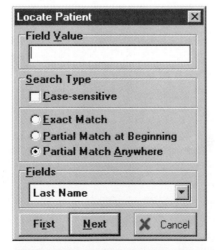

Figure 7-16 Locate Patient dialog box.

entered in the Field Value box if they appear anywhere in the item. For example, if "son" were entered in the Field Value box, the system would return entries such as "Masterson," "Sonya," "Wilson's Hardware," and so on.

Fields   Searches can be conducted on a variety of different fields of information, including last name, Social Security number, ZIP Code, chart number, assigned provider, and so on. The specific box of information is selected from the choices in the Fields drop-down list.

First   When the First button is clicked, the system locates the first patient that matches the search criteria and displays that patient's Transaction Entry dialog box. For example, if a search were conducted for patient's of Dr. Yan, clicking the First button would display the Transaction Entry dialog box for the first patient (in order of chart numbers) who has Dr. Yan as his or her assigned provider.

Next   When the Next button is clicked, the system locates the next patient who matches the criteria and displays his or her Transaction Entry dialog box.

Cancel   When the Cancel button is clicked, the search is terminated and the Locate Patient dialog box is closed.

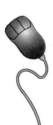

Exercise 7-8

Using the two Locate buttons, find transactions for Samuel Bell.

MediSoft Program Date: March 3, 2003.

1. Open the Transaction Entry dialog box.

2. Click the top Locate button. The Locate Patient dialog box is displayed.

3. In the Field Value box, key *Bell*.

4. Click the radio button for Exact Match.

5. Accept the default entry of "Last Name" in the Fields text box.

6. Click the First button to begin the search.

7. The Transaction Entry dialog box for Herbert Bell, the first "Bell" in the database when sorting alphabetically by last and then first name, is displayed.

8. Click the bottom Locate button to find the next patient with the last name of Bell.

9. The Transaction Entry dialog box for Janine Bell is displayed. Click the bottom Locate button until BELLSAMØ (Samuel Bell) is listed in the Chart box. Press the Enter key to display Samuel Bell's transactions.

10. Close the Transaction Entry dialog box.

ADDITIONAL INFORMATION IN THE TRANSACTION ENTRY DIALOG BOX

The Transaction Entry dialog box also includes other useful information. This data cannot be edited but provides valuable information about a patient and a patient's account. This information is listed in four sections in the Transaction Entry dialog box.

DIAGNOSIS

The top right side of the dialog box displays a patient's diagnosis. There are boxes for up to four diagnoses (see Figure 7-17).

DIAG 1, 2, 3, 4   The system copies a patient's diagnosis information from the case file and displays it in the DIAG 1, 2, 3, or 4 box.

INSURANCE CARRIER/ GUARANTOR FINANCIAL RESPONSIBILITY

The section on the left side of the dialog box displays information about the financial responsibilities of the guarantor and the insurance carrier. An estimate of the portion of a bill that will be paid by an insurance carrier(s) is listed, followed by the amount the guarantor is responsible for paying (see Figure 7-18).

Policy 1, Policy 2, Policy 3   A patient's insurance carriers are listed in the Policy 1, Policy 2, and Policy 3 boxes. To the right of the insurance policy is a column labeled "Est. Resp." This is the dollar amount of the estimated responsibility for each insurance carrier.

Guarantor   The system automatically calculates the dollar amount that the guarantor is responsible for paying, after deducting the estimated amount paid by the insurance carrier. This amount is listed in the Guarantor box followed by the guarantor's last name and first name.

Policy Copay   The Policy Copay box lists the amount of a patient's copayment, if applicable.

OA   The Other Arrangements box indicates whether special conditions have been set up for a patient's billing. The system automatically enters information recorded in the Other Arrangements box in the Account tab of the Case dialog box.

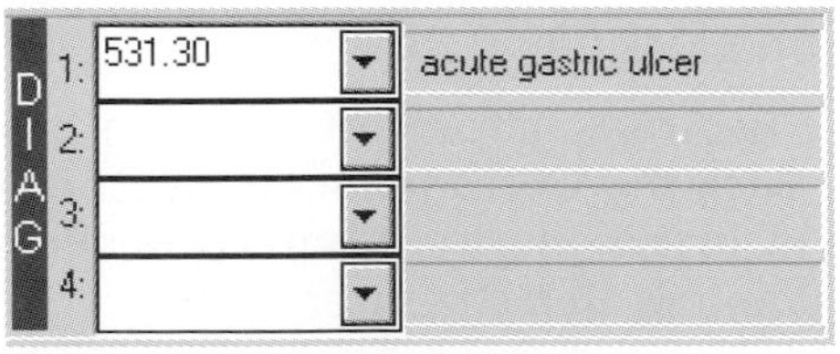

Figure 7-17 Diagnosis information.

	Est. Resp.
Policy 1: Champ VA	20.00
Policy 2:	0.00
Policy 3:	0.00
Guarantor: Fitzwilliams, John	5.00
Policy Copay:	OA:

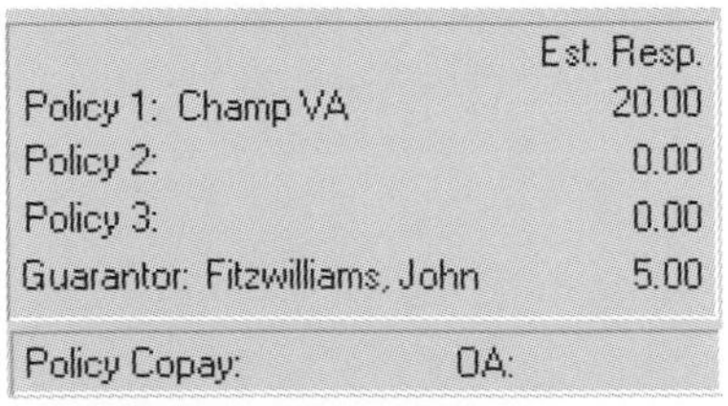

Figure 7-18 Financial Responsibility information.

LAST VISIT AND LAST PAYMENT   The middle section of the dialog box lists information about the patient's most recent visit and most recent payment (see Figure 7-19).

Last Visit   The Date box within the Last Visit area lists the date of a patient's most recent visit to a particular physician. The Visit box lists the visit series information as entered in the Account tab of the Case dialog box. The Visit box can be edited from within the Transaction Entry dialog box.

Last Payment   The Last Payment area lists the date (Date box) and the amount of the last payment received (Amount box) on a patient's account.

ACCOUNT SUMMARY   The right side of the dialog box contains a summary of a patient's account, including charges, adjustments, and payments, for an active case (see Figure 7-20).

Charges   The Charges box lists the total of the charges for a particular case.

Adjustments   The Adjustments box lists the total of the adjustments for this case.

Sub Total   The Sub Total box lists a subtotal of the amounts shown in the Charges and Adjustments boxes. If the amount in the Adjustments box is preceded by a minus sign, that amount is subtracted from the amount in the Charges box.

Payment   The Payment box lists the total payments received to date for this case.

Balance   The Balance box lists the amount due.

Account Total   The Account Total box lists the total amount owed for a particular patient for all cases, not just the case that is displayed in the Case box.

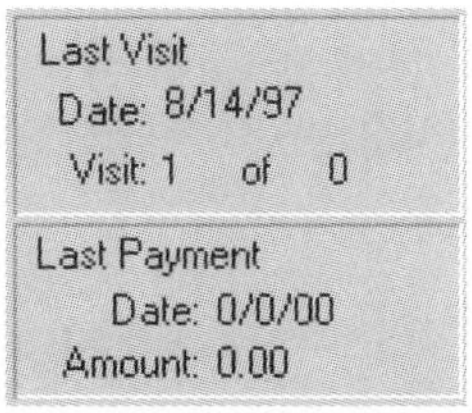

Last Visit
Date: 8/14/97
Visit: 1   of   0

Last Payment
Date: 0/0/00
Amount: 0.00

Figure 7-19 Last Visit information.

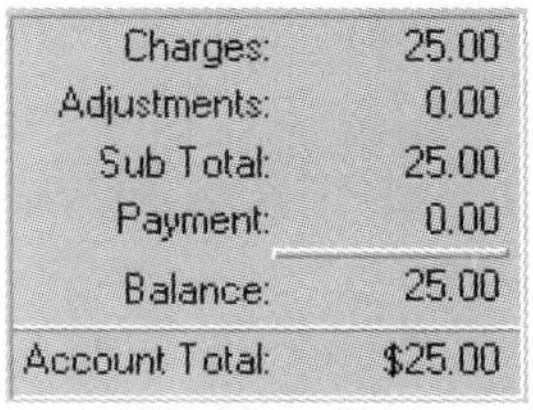

Charges:	25.00
Adjustments:	0.00
Sub Total:	25.00
Payment:	0.00
Balance:	25.00
Account Total:	$25.00

Figure 7-20 Account Summary information.

CHAPTER REVIEW

USING TERMINOLOGY

Match the terms on the left with the definitions on the right.

_____ **1.** adjustments

_____ **2.** charges

_____ **3.** modifiers

_____ **4.** MultiLink codes

_____ **5.** payments

a. One- or two-digit codes that add a specific description to a procedure code.

b. Changes to patients' accounts.

c. The amounts billed by a provider for particular services.

d. Monies paid to a medical practice by patients and insurance carriers.

e. Groups of procedure code entries that are related to a single activity.

CHECKING YOUR UNDERSTANDING

Answer the questions below in the space provided.

6. Why is it important that the document number entered in the Payment tab match the document number of the charge being paid?

_____

_____

7. List two advantages of using MultiLink codes.

_____

_____

8. If a patient is paying by check, what should be entered in the Description box on the Payment tab?

_____

_____

9. What date should be entered in the Dates boxes on the Charge tab?

_____

_____

10. When entering an adjustment that will reduce the balance owed by a patient, what must be done to indicate that it is a reduction?

_____

_____

11. What is the Transaction Documentation feature used for?

_____

_____

12. An established patient of Dr. Yan comes in for an emergency visit but cannot get an appointment with Dr. Yan. Instead, she sees Dr. Jessica Rudner. When entering the charge for the visit, how would you indicate that the patient saw Dr. Rudner and not Dr. Yan for that particular office visit?

_____

_____

APPLYING KNOWLEDGE

Answer the questions below in the space provided.

13. After you have entered a payment for $20, you realize it should have been $30. What should you do?

_____

_____

_____

14. The receptionist working at the front desk phones to tell you that Maritza Ramos has just seen the physician and would like to know before she leaves the office whether her insurance carrier has paid anything on her January 14, 2003 office visit. You are in the middle of entering an insurance payment for another patient. What should you do first? What is your reasoning?

_____

_____

_____

AT THE COMPUTER

Answer the following questions at the computer:

15. Conduct a search for transactions for Randall Klein that occurred on March 3, 2003. List the procedure codes and charges for those transactions.

16. Today is December 8, 2003. A check for $100 arrives from Blue Cross/Blue Shield as payment for James Smith's facial-nerve function studies performed on May 20, 2003. The check number is 49703024. Enter the payment, and apply it to the charge. Save the transaction. What is the remaining amount of the charge that is James Smith's responsibility to pay?

17. Enter a charge transaction for the annual exam case for Samuel Bell, which occurred on November 18, 2002. The procedure code is 99396. Save the charge transaction. On November 18, Samuel's father pays the amount that is the guarantor's responsibility. Locate this amount in the Transaction Entry dialog box, and enter the payment, which is made by Check Number 1049. Save the payment transaction. Three weeks later, a check comes from East Ohio PPO, Samuel's insurance carrier. This check is in the amount of $104 and is Check Number 3394567. Enter this payment, and save the payment transaction.

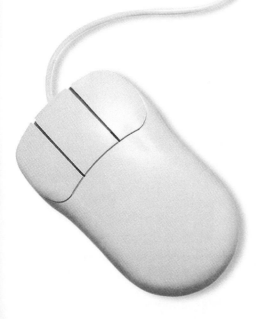

CHAPTER 8 Scheduling

WHAT YOU NEED TO KNOW

To use this chapter, you need to know how to:

◆ Start MediSoft, use menus, and enter and edit text.
◆ Work with chart numbers and codes.

OBJECTIVES

In this chapter, you will learn how to:

◆ Start Office Hours.
◆ View the appointment schedule.
◆ Enter an appointment.
◆ Change or delete an appointment.
◆ Move or copy an appointment.
◆ Search for an existing appointment.
◆ Create a recall list.
◆ Enter a break in a provider's schedule.

KEY TERMS

Office Hours break
Office Hours schedule

INTRODUCTION TO OFFICE HOURS

Appointment scheduling is one of the most important tasks in a medical office. Different procedures take different lengths of time, and each appointment must be the right length. On the one hand, physicians want to be able to go from one appointment to another without unnecessary breaks in between patients. On the other hand, patients should not be kept waiting more than a few minutes for a physician. Managing and juggling the schedule is usually the job of a medical office assistant working at the front desk. MediSoft provides a special program to handle appointment scheduling, called Office Hours.

OVERVIEW OF THE OFFICE HOURS SCREEN

The Office Hours program has its own menu bar and toolbar. The Office Hours menu bar lists the menus available: File, Edit, Search, List, Tools, and Help (see Figure 8-1). Under the menu bar is a toolbar with shortcut buttons. The functions of Office Hours are accessed by selecting a choice from one of the menus or by clicking a shortcut button (see Figure 8-2).

Located just below the menu bar, the toolbar contains a series of buttons that represent the most common activities performed in Office Hours. These buttons are shortcuts for frequently used menu commands. The toolbar displays 11 buttons (see Figure 8-2 and Table 8-1.)

The left half of the Office Hours screen displays the current date and a calendar of the current month (see Figure 8-3 on page 148). The current date is highlighted on the calendar. Clicking a different date on the calendar switches the schedule on the right side of the screen to the new day. Clicking the Go to Today shortcut button, shown in Figure 8-2, resets the screen back to the current date (the Windows System Date.)

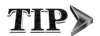

The Office Hours program uses the Windows System Date as the default date. If you want the default date to be different from the current date, the Windows System Date must be changed *before* Office Hours is started.

Figure 8-1 Office Hours menu bar.

Go to Today
shortcut button

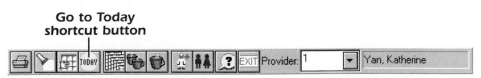

Figure 8-2 Office Hours toolbar.

Table 8-1   **Office Hours Toolbar Buttons**

Button	Button Name	Associated Function	Activity
	Print Report	Report printing	Print current day's schedule.
	Find Appointment	Find Appointment dialog box	Search for existing appointments.
	Go to Date	Go to Date dialog box	Choose any date as the current date.
	Go to Today	Displays current date	Return the calendar date to the current date.
	Repeating Appointments	Repeating Appointments dialog box	Allow scheduling of multiple appointments for a patient.
	Recurring Breaks	Recurring Breaks dialog box	Create breaks to occur at regular intervals.
	Create a Break	Creates break	Create breaks one at a time.
	Provider List	Provider List dialog box	Add, edit, or delete providers.
	Patient List	Patient List dialog box	Add, edit, or delete patients.
	Show/Hide Hints	Balloon Help	Turn the Hints feature on or off.
	Exit Program	Exit	Exit the Office Hours program.

Office Hours schedule *a listing of time slots for a particular day for a specific provider.*

The **Office Hours schedule**, shown on the right half of the screen, is a listing of time slots for a particular day for a specific provider. The provider's name and number is displayed at the top. The provider can be easily changed by clicking the triangle button in the Provider box. When a time slot is clicked on the schedule, the cursor moves to the name box in the appointment area of the screen (at the lower left). When a patient's name is entered in the Name box, it is automatically entered in the slot that is highlighted on the schedule.

PROGRAM OPTIONS

When Office Hours is installed in a medical practice, it is set up to reflect the needs of that particular practice. Most offices which have MediSoft already have Office Hours set up and running. However, if it is just being installed, the options to set up the Office Hours pro-

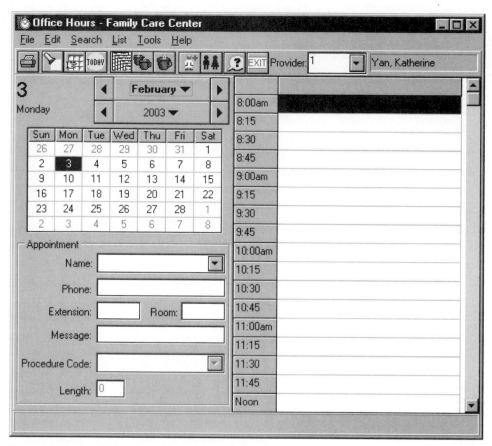

Figure 8-3 The Office Hours screen.

gram can be found in the Program Options dialog box, which is accessed by clicking Program Options on the Office Hours File menu. The Program Options dialog box provides a number of setup options, including a feature that allows more than one patient to be scheduled in the same time slot.

ENTERING AND EXITING OFFICE HOURS

Office Hours can be started from within MediSoft or directly from Windows 95. To access Office Hours from within MediSoft, Appointment Book is clicked on the Activities menu. Office Hours can also be started by clicking the corresponding shortcut button on the toolbar.

Office Hours shortcut button.

To start Office Hours without entering MediSoft first:

1. Click the Start button on the Windows 95 task bar.
2. Click MediSoft on the Program submenu.
3. Click Office Hours on the MediSoft submenu.

The Office Hours program is closed by clicking Exit on the Office Hours File menu, or by clicking the Exit button on its toolbar. If Office Hours was started from within MediSoft, exiting will return you to MediSoft. If Office Hours was started directly from Windows 95, clicking Exit will return you to the Windows 95 desktop.

ENTERING APPOINTMENTS

Entering an appointment begins with selecting the provider for whom the appointment is being scheduled. The current provider is listed in the Provider box at the top right of the screen (see Figure 8-4). Clicking the triangle button displays a drop-down list of providers in the system. To choose a different provider, click the name of the provider on the drop-down list.

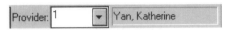

Figure 8-4 Provider box.

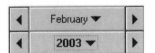

Figure 8-5 Month and Year triangle buttons.

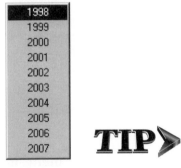

Figure 8-6 Year drop-down list.

After the provider is selected, the date of the desired appointment must be chosen. Dates are changed by clicking the Month and Year triangle buttons and then clicking the date on the calendar (see Figure 8-5). The Year drop-down list displays ten years at a time (see Figure 8-6). Suppose, for example, that a patient needs an appointment on January 17, 2003. January is selected from the list of months on the Month drop-down list, and 2003 is selected from the list of years on the Year drop-down list. The date is selected by clicking 17 on the calendar. After the provider and date have been selected, patient information is entered into various boxes in the appointment area of the screen (see Figure 8-7). In Office Hours, the Tab key is used to enter information and to move from box to box.

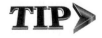

If the desired year is not on the Year drop-down list, click the first entry (to see prior years) or the last entry (to see future years). Then click the Year button again to display additional years.

The month and year can also be changed by clicking the triangle buttons that appear to the right and left of the Month and Year buttons. Clicking the triangle button to the left of the Month button displays the prior month; clicking the triangle button to the left of the Year button displays the prior year. Clicking twice on the buttons displays two months ago and two years ago, respectively. In similar fashion, the triangle buttons on the right are used for moving ahead in time, one for the month and one for the year.

If the date is being changed by more than one or two months or years, it is faster to use the Month and Year buttons to make a selection. Using these buttons, only two clicks are required. To select a date six months ahead with the right triangle button requires six clicks.

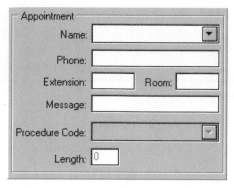

Figure 8-7 Appointment area of the Office Hours screen.

Name   A patient's name is selected from the drop-down list in the Name box. An alternative method is to enter the first few letters of the patient's chart number in the Name box. The program then displays a drop-down list, and the chart number that is highlighted can be accepted or another patient can be selected by clicking a different chart number. However, when this latter method is used, the program may not automatically display the patient's phone number. For this reason, you may wish to select a patient by clicking his or her name on the drop-down list.

Phone   After a name is selected from the Name drop-down list, that patient's phone number is automatically entered in the Phone box.

Extension   If there is a phone extension, it is listed automatically when a patient is selected in the Name box.

Room   The number of the room reserved for a particular patient can be entered in the Room box.

Message   Any special information about an appointment is entered in the Message box.

Procedure Code   If the procedure code is known, it is entered in the Procedure Code box by making a selection from the drop-down list of codes or keying the code.

Length   The amount of time an appointment will take (minutes) is entered in the Length box. If an appointment is more than 15 minutes, the time slots below the first 15-minute slot on the schedule will be shaded. The shading indicates that those time slots are being used by the patient listed in the slot immediately above the shading.

After the boxes on the left side of the screen have been completed, pressing the Tab key enters the information on the schedule. The patient's name appears in the time slot corresponding to the appointment time.

LOOKING FOR A FUTURE DATE

Go to Date shortcut button.

Often a patient will need a follow-up appointment at a certain time in the future. For example, suppose a physician has seen a certain patient on a particular day and would like a checkup appointment in three weeks. The most efficient way to search for a future appointment in Office Hours is to use the Go to Date shortcut button on the toolbar. (This feature can also be accessed on the Edit menu.)

Clicking the Go to Date shortcut button displays the Go to Date dialog box (see Figure 8-8). Within the dialog box, five boxes offer options for choosing a future date.

Go to __ this Date   This box is used to locate an appointment on a specific date. For example, if a patient needs an appointment on October 20, 2003, that date would be entered in this box.

Go to __ DAYS From the Current Date   This box is used to locate a date a specific number of days in the future. For example, if a patient needs an appointment 10 days from the current day, "10" would be entered in this box.

Go to __ WEEKS From the Current Week   This box is used when a patient needs an appointment a specific number of weeks in the future, such as six weeks from the current day.

Go to __ MONTHS From the Current Month   This box is used when a patient needs an appointment a specific number of months in the future, such as three months from the current day.

Go to __ YEARS From the Current Year   Similar to the weeks and months options, this box is used when an appointment is needed in one, or several years in the future.

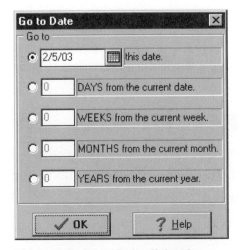

Figure 8-8 Go to Date dialog box.

All dates entered in the Go to Date dialog box should be entered in the MMDDCCYY format. For example, February 3, 2003, would be entered as "02032003." If dates are not entered in this format, the program will assume the dates are in the twentieth century, not the twenty-first century. For example, if the entry were "020303," (the MMDDYY format), the program would display the schedule for February 3, 1903, not February 3, 2003.

After a future date option has been selected, clicking the OK button begins the search. The system locates the future date and displays the schedule for that date.

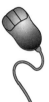

Exercise 8-1

Enter an appointment with Dr. John Rudner at 2:30 p.m. next Monday for Herbert Bell. The appointment is 15 minutes in length.

Windows System Date: February 3, 2003

1. Start MediSoft. Change the Windows System Date. Start Office Hours by clicking the Office Hours shortcut button on the toolbar.

2. Click John Rudner on the drop-down list in the Provider box.

3. Click next Monday on the calendar.

4. In the schedule, click the 2:30 p.m. time slot. (You will need to use the scroll bar to view 2:30 p.m.) The Appointment area of the window is now ready to accept data on the patient.

5. Click Herbert Bell from the list of names on the drop-down list in the Name box. The system automatically fills in the Phone box. Herbert Bell's name is displayed in the 2:30 p.m. time slot on the schedule.

6. Verify that the time displayed in the Length box is 15 minutes. Press the Tab key.

 TIP At the *end* of each exercise in this chapter, except Exercise 8-11, you should click the Go to Today shortcut button. This action resets the Office Hours calendar to the current date (February 3, 2003) in preparation for the next exercise.

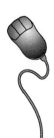

Exercise 8-2

Enter the following appointments with Dr. John Rudner:

Next Monday at 3:15 p.m. for John Fitzwilliams, 30 minutes in length.

Windows System Date: February 3, 2003

1. Verify that "2 Rudner, John" is displayed in the Provider box.

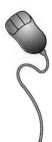

2. Click the Go to Date shortcut button. Click the Go to __ WEEKS From the Current Week radio button. Key *1* in the box. Click the OK button. Verify that February 10, 2003 is highlighted on the calendar.

3. In the schedule, click the 3:15 p.m. time-slot box.

4. Click John Fitzwilliams on the Names drop-down list.

5. Press the Tab key until the cursor is in the Length box.

6. Key *30* in the Length box.

7. Press the Tab key.

8. Click the Go to Today shortcut button to reset the calendar to February 3, 2003.

9. Enter an appointment on next Monday at 3:45 p.m. for Leila Patterson, 15 minutes in length.

10. Click the Go to Today shortcut button.

11. Enter an appointment on next Tuesday at 12:15 p.m. for James Smith, 30 minutes in length.

12. Use Office Hours' Go to Date feature to schedule an appointment two weeks later for James Smith at 12:15 p.m., 15 minutes in length.

Exercise 8-3

Enter the following appointments with Dr. Jessica Rudner.

Windows System Date: February 3, 2003

1. Click Dr. Jessica Rudner from the list of providers in the Provider drop-down list.

2. Enter an appointment for next Monday at 2:00 p.m. for Janine Bell, 15 minutes in length.

3. Click the Go to Today shortcut button to reset the calendar to February 3, 2003.

4. Use Office Hours' Go to Date feature to schedule an appointment three weeks from the current date at 1:15 p.m. for Sarina Bell, 30 minutes in length.

5. Click the Go to Today shortcut button.

6. Use the Go to Date feature to schedule an appointment for Sarah Fitzwilliams. Make the appointment two days from today at 9:00 a.m., 60 minutes in length.

7. Temporarily leave Office Hours by clicking the minimize button in the upper right corner of the window.

Exercise 8-4

Enter an appointment with Dr. Katherine Yan at 9:15 a.m. this Thursday for John Gardiner, 30 minutes in length.

Windows System Date: February 3, 2003

1. Go to the Transaction Entry dialog box.

2. Click John Gardiner as the patient.

3. Click the Office Hours button on the Windows 95 task bar (bottom of screen). Notice that the Transaction Entry dialog box is still partially visible underneath the Office Hours window.

4. Enter the appointment.

5. Exit Office Hours.

6. In MediSoft, close the Transaction Entry dialog box.

SEARCHING FOR AVAILABLE APPOINTMENT TIME

Often it is necessary to search for available appointment space on a particular day and at a specific time. For example, a patient needs a 30-minute appointment and would like it to be during lunch hour, which is from 12:00 p.m. to 1:00 p.m. He can only get away from the office on Mondays and Fridays. The Office Hours Search feature makes it easy to locate an appointment slot that meets these requirements.

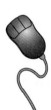

Exercise 8-5

Search for the next available appointment slot in Office Hours.

Windows System Date: February 3, 2003

1. Start Office Hours. Click Dr. Jessica Rudner on the drop-down list in the Provider box.

2. On the Search menu, click Find. The Find Available Appointment Spaces dialog box is displayed (see Figure 8-9).

3. Key *45* in the Appointment Length Wanted box. Press the Tab key. Appointments can be from 5 minutes to 120 minutes in length.

4. Key *10* in the Beginning Time box and click the Am radio button if it is not already selected.

5. Key *4* in the Ending Time box and click the Pm radio button if it is not already selected.

6. To search for an appointment on Tuesday or Thursday, click the Sunday, Monday, Wednesday, Friday, and Saturday boxes to deselect those days of the week. Check marks should only appear in the Tuesday and Thursday boxes.

7. Click the Search button to begin looking for an appointment slot. The system locates the first available slot that meets these specifications and highlights that slot on the schedule (see Figure 8-10).

8. Click **Juanita Ramos** on the drop-down list in the Name box.

9. Press the **Tab** key until the cursor is in the Length box.

10. Key *45* and press the **Tab** key.

11. Verify that the appointment has been entered by looking at the schedule.

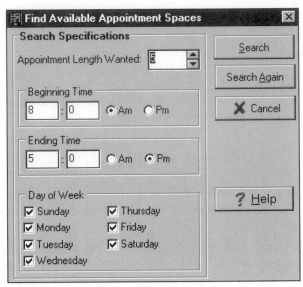

Figure 8-9 Find Available Appointment Spaces dialog box.

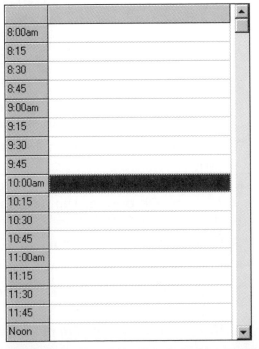

Figure 8-10 Schedule with available slot highlighted.

Exercise 8-6

Schedule Randall Klein for a 60-minute appointment with Dr. John Rudner. Mr. Klein is only available between 11:00 a.m. and 2:00 p.m.

Windows System Date: February 3, 2003

1. Click the desired provider in the Provider box.

2. Click Find on the Search menu to display the Find Available Appointment Spaces dialog box.

3. In the Appointment Length Wanted box, use the triangle buttons to select 60.

4. Key *11* in the Beginning Time box.

5. Key *2* in the Ending Time box.

6. In the Day of Week box, select all the days except Saturday and Sunday.

7. Click the Search button. The first available slot that meets the requirements is highlighted on the schedule.

8. Click once in the slot to activate the Appointment information.

9. Click Randall Klein from the drop-down list in the Name box.

10. Key *60* in the Length box, and press the Tab key. The appointment is entered on the schedule.

Exercise 8-7

Schedule Juanita Ramos for a 30-minute appointment with Dr. Jessica Rudner six months from the current date. Ms. Ramos is available after 3:00 p.m. any weekday except Wednesday.

Windows System Date: February 3, 2003

1. Click the desired provider in the Provider box.

2. Click Go to Date on the Edit menu or click the Go to Date shortcut button. The Go to Date dialog box is displayed.

3. Click the Go to ___ Months From the Current Month radio button.

4. Key *6* in the Go to ___ MONTHS From the Current Month box. Click the OK button. The new date is displayed on the calendar and schedule. Notice that August 3, 2003, is a Sunday.

5. Click Find on the Search menu.

6. Key *30* in the Appointment Length Wanted box.

7. Key *3* and click the Pm radio button in the Beginning Time box.

8. Key *4:45* and click the Pm radio button in the Ending Time box.

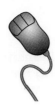

9. In the Day of Week box, click **Monday, Tuesday, Thursday, and Friday.**

10. Click the **Search button.**

11. Enter an appointment for Ms. Ramos in the first available slot that meets her requirements.

BOOKING REPEATED APPOINTMENTS

Repeating Appointments shortcut button.

Some patients require appointments on a repeated basis, such as every Thursday for eight weeks. Repeated appointments are set up by clicking Repeating Appointments on the Edit menu or by clicking the Repeating Appointments shortcut button. The Repeating Appointments dialog box provides a number of choices for setting up repeating appointments (see Figure 8-11).

The top section of the dialog box contains information about the appointment. The day of the week and the number of weeks for which an appointment is needed are selected. The starting date and time are entered.

The lower half of the dialog box lists information about the patient. The boxes in this area are identical to those used when entering a standard appointment. When a patient is selected from the drop-down list in the Name box, the system automatically completes the Phone and Extension boxes. If there is no extension, the box will remain blank. Information about the appointment can be entered in the Message box. If the CPT code is known, it can be selected from the drop-down list in the Procedure Code box. The length of the appointment is specified in the Length box.

When all the information is complete, the OK button is clicked. The repeated appointments now are displayed on the schedule.

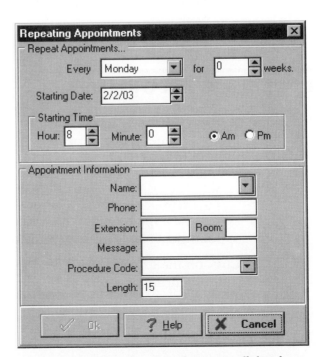

Figure 8-11 Repeating Appointments dialog box.

Exercise 8-8

Schedule Li Y Wong for a 15-minute appointment with Dr. Katherine Yan, once a week for six weeks. Mrs. Wong has requested that the appointments be at the same time every week, preferably in the early morning.

Windows System Date: February 3, 2003

1. Click the desired provider on the Provider drop-down list.

2. Click Repeating Appointments on the Edit menu to display the Repeating Appointments dialog box or click the Repeating Appointments shortcut button.

3. In the Every box, accept the default entry of Monday.

4. Key 6 for the number of weeks.

5. In the Starting Date box, click the triangle buttons until "2/10/03" is displayed, which is one week from the current date.

6. Accept the default entry of 8:00 a.m. in the Starting Time box.

7. Click Li Y Wong on the Name drop-down list.

8. Click the OK button.

9. Click February 10, 2003, to verify that Mrs. Wong is scheduled for an appointment at 8:00 a.m.

10. Check one or two of the other five dates to verify that Mrs. Wong is also scheduled on these days.

CHANGING OR DELETING APPOINTMENTS

Very often it is necessary to change a patient's appointment or cancel an appointment. Changing an appointment is accomplished with the Cut and Paste commands on the Office Hours Edit menu.

The following steps are used to reschedule an appointment:

1. Locate the appointment that needs to be changed. Make sure the appointment slot is visible on the schedule.

2. Click on the existing time-slot box. A grey border surrounds the slot to indicate it is selected.

3. Click Cut on the Edit menu. The appointment disappears from the schedule.

4. Click the date on the calendar when the appointment is to be rescheduled.

5. Click on the desired time-slot box on the schedule. The slot becomes active.

6. Click Paste on the Edit menu. The patient's name appears in the new time-slot box.

The following steps are used to cancel an appointment without rescheduling:

1. Locate the appointment on the schedule.

2. Click on the time-slot box to select the appointment.

3. Click Cut on the Edit menu. The appointment disappears from the schedule.

Exercise 8-9

Change Janine Bell's and John Gardiner's appointments.

Windows System Date: February 3, 2003

1. Click Jessica Rudner on the Provider box drop-down list.

2. Click Monday, February 10, 2003, on the calendar.

3. Locate Janine Bell's 2:00 p.m. appointment on the schedule. Click the 2:00 p.m. time-slot box.

4. Click Cut on the Edit menu. Janine Bell's appointment is removed from the 2:00 p.m. time-slot box.

5. Click the 3:00 p.m. time-slot box.

6. Click Paste on the Edit menu. Janine Bell's name is displayed in the 3:00 p.m. time-slot box.

7. Click Katherine Yan on the Provider drop-down list.

8. Click Thursday, February 6, 2003, on the calendar.

9. Locate John Gardiner's 9:15 a.m. appointment. Remove his appointment from the 9:15 a.m. time slot.

10. Click Friday, February 7, 2003, on the calendar.

11. Enter John Gardiner's appointment in the 9:15 a.m. time slot.

12. Exit Office Hours.

CREATING A RECALL LIST

Medical offices frequently must keep track of patients who need to return for a future appointment. Some offices schedule future appointments when the patient is leaving the office. For example, if a patient has just seen a physician and needs to return for a follow-up appointment in six weeks, the appointment is usually made before the patient leaves the office. However, when the appointment is needed some time further in the future, such as one year later, it is not always practical to set the appointment so far in advance. It is difficult for the patient and for the physician to know their schedules a year in advance. For this reason, many offices keep a list of patients who need to be contacted for a future appointment.

In MediSoft, a recall list can be created and maintained by clicking Patient Recall on the Lists menu. Patients can also be added to the recall list by clicking the Patient Recall Entry shortcut button on the toolbar. When Patient Recall is selected from the Lists menu, the Patient Recall List dialog box is displayed (see Figure 8-12). This dialog box organizes the recall information in a column format. The scroll bar is used to display the last three columns on the right.

- **Date of Recall**   Lists the date for which the recall is scheduled for.
- **Name**   Displays the patient's name.
- **Phone**   Lists the patient's phone number, making it easy to call patients for appointments without having to look up the phone number in another dialog box.
- **Status**   Indicates the patient's recall status: Call, Call again, Appointment, No appointment.
- **Provider**   Displays the provider code for the patient's provider.

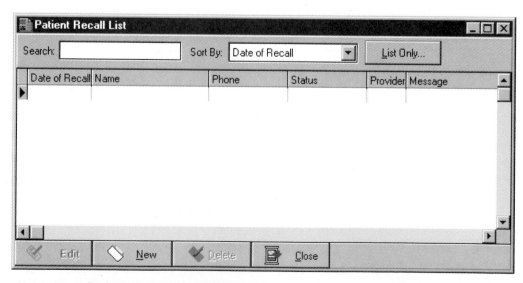

Figure 8-12 Patient Recall List dialog box.

◆ **Message**   Displays the entry made in the Message box of the Patient Recall dialog box.

◆ **Extension**   Lists the patient's phone extension.

◆ **Chart Number**   Displays the patient's chart number.

◆ **Procedure Code**   Lists the procedure code for the procedure for which the patient is being recalled.

The Patient Recall List dialog box contains the following boxes:

Search   The Search box is used to locate a specific patient on the recall list. Entering the first few letters or numbers in the Search box displays the selection that is the closest match to the search criteria.

Sort By   The choices in the Sort By box determine whether patients are listed in the dialog box by Date of Recall, Chart Number, or Provider. The default entry is Date of Recall.

The Patient Recall List dialog box also contains these buttons: List Only, Edit, New, Delete, and Close.

List Only   The List Only button is used to select temporarily the list of patients who are on the recall list in the Patient Recall List dialog box. When the List Only button is clicked, the List Only Recalls That Match dialog box is displayed with five radio buttons that correspond to the patient's recall status: Call, Call Again, Appointment Set, No Appointment, and All. The latter is used to select all patients regardless of recall status. For example, if the Call radio button is selected, the dialog box lists only those patients who require phone calls. To apply the option selected, the OK button is clicked and the revised list of patients is displayed in the Patient Recall List dialog box. Data on the other patients are not deleted, just temporarily hidden from view. To see the full list of patients, reenter the List Only Recalls That Match dialog box by clicking the List Only button, click the All radio button, and click the OK button.

Edit   Clicking the Edit button displays the Patient Recall dialog box for the patient whose entry is highlighted. The information on the patient can then be edited by making different selections in the boxes.

New   Clicking the New button displays an empty Patient Recall dialog box, in which data on a new recall patient can be entered.

Delete   Clicking the Delete button deletes from the patient recall list data on the patient whose entry is highlighted.

Close   The Close button is used to exit the Patient Recall List dialog box.

ADDING A PATIENT TO THE RECALL LIST

Patient Recall Entry shortcut button.

Patients are added to the recall list by clicking the New button in the Patient Recall List dialog box or by clicking the Patient Recall Entry shortcut button. When either of these actions is performed, the Patient Recall dialog box is displayed (see Figure 8-13). The Patient Recall dialog box contains the following boxes:

Recall Date The date a patient needs to return to see a physician is entered in the Recall Date box in MMDDYY format.

Provider A patient's provider is selected from the drop-down list.

Chart A patient's chart number is selected from the drop-down list, or the first few letters of a patient's chart number are entered in the Chart box.

Name, Phone, Extension After a chart number is entered, the system automatically completes the Name, Phone, and Extension boxes.

Procedure If the procedure for which a patient is returning is known, it is entered in the Procedure box in one of two ways. The procedure code can be selected from the drop-down list, or the first few numbers can be entered and the system will display on the drop-down list the entry that most closely matches the entered numbers. This is especially valuable in practices in which there are hundreds of procedure codes, because it eliminates the need to scroll through several hundred codes to locate the desired one.

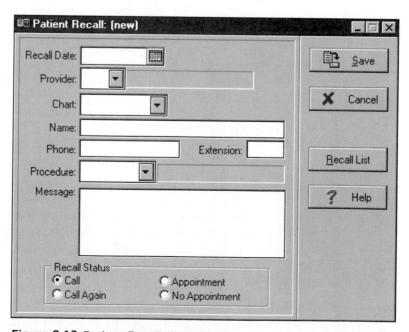

Figure 8-13 Patient Recall dialog box.

Message The Message box is used to record any special notes, reminders, or instructions about a patient and his or her appointment.

Recall Status The choices in the Recall Status box are used to indicate the action that needs to be taken. They include:

Call The Call button is used when a patient needs to be telephoned regarding a future appointment.

Call Again The Call Again button is used when a patient has been called once, but contact was not made and an additional call is necessary.

Appointment The Appointment button is used when a patient has an appointment already scheduled.

No Appointment The No Appointment button is used when a patient has been contacted for an appointment but has declined for some reason.

After the information has been entered in the dialog box, clicking the Save button saves the data and adds the patient to the recall list. In addition to the Save button, the Patient Recall dialog box contains these buttons: Cancel, Recall List, and Help. The Cancel button exits the dialog box without saving the data entered. The Recall List button in the Patient Recall dialog box is used to display the Patient Recall List dialog box. The Help button displays MediSoft's online help for the Patient Recall dialog box.

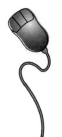

Exercise 8-10

John Fitzwilliams needs to receive a phone call one year from today to set up an appointment for Procedure 99396, established patient, 40-64 years, periodic preventive medicine. Add John Fitzwilliams to the recall list.

Windows System Date: February 3, 2003

1. Click the Patient Recall Entry shortcut button. The Patient Recall dialog box is displayed.

2. In the Recall Date box, enter February 3, 2004, in MMDDYY format.

3. Determine which physician is John Fitzwilliams's provider. (Look in the Patient/Guarantor dialog box for this information.)

4. Click John Fitzwilliams's provider on the drop-down list in the Provider box.

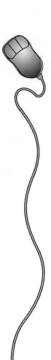

5. Enter John Fitzwilliams's chart number in the Chart box by keying the first few letters of his chart number. Notice that the system automatically completes the Phone box. (The Extension box would also be completed if there were an extension).

6. Enter the procedure code in the Procedure box by keying *99396* (established patient, 40-64 years, periodic preventive medicine).

7. In the Message box, key *Was changing jobs; ask about new insurance coverage.*

8. Verify that the Call radio button in the Recall Status box is selected.

9. Click the Save button to save the entry.

10. Click Patient Recall on the Lists menu.

11. Verify that the entry for John Fitzwilliams has been added to the recall list.

12. Close the Patient Recall List dialog box.

CREATING BREAKS

Office Hours break a block of time when a physician is unavailable for appointments with patients.

Office Hours provides features for inserting standard breaks in providers' schedules. The **Office Hours break** is a block of time when a physician is unavailable for appointments with patients. Standard breaks included in Office Hours are Lunch, Meeting, Personal, Emergency, Break, Vacation, Seminar, Holiday, Trip, and Surgery. In Office Hours, breaks can be created one at a time or on a recurring basis for all providers. One-time breaks, such as those for a vacation, are best entered using the Create Break command. The Create a Recurring Break command is useful for entering lunch hours, providers' days off, staff meetings, and other events that occur frequently and with some regularity.

CREATE BREAK COMMAND

Often breaks need to be inserted into a provider's schedule when he or she is not available for appointments with patients. For example, if a physician will be in surgery on Thursday from 9 a.m. until 12:00 p.m., that time period must be marked as unavailable on his or her schedule. This is accomplished by using the Create Break command.

Create Break shortcut button.

To set up a break for a current provider (that is, the provider listed in the Office Hours Provider box), click Create Break on the Edit menu or click the Create a Break shortcut button. This action causes a group of break buttons to appear in the lower left area of the window (see Figure 8-14). To create a break, click one of the buttons (surgery, for example), and then click the time-slot box in the schedule where the

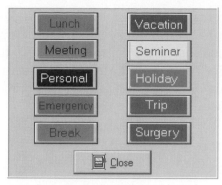

Figure 8-14 Break buttons.

break will occur. The time slot then displays the name of the break button that was selected. If a break extends over more than one time slot, additional breaks can be added by holding down the mouse button and dragging through the additional slots. If a break needs to be moved or deleted, the Break feature must be closed first and then the Cut and Paste commands are used. To exit the Break feature, click the Close button displayed underneath the break buttons.

Exercise 8-11

Dr. Jessica Rudner will be away at a seminar from Monday, February 17, 2003 to Wednesday, February 19, 2003. Enter this as a break on her schedule.

Windows System Date: February 3, 2003

1. Start Office Hours.

2. Check that Dr. Jessica Rudner is the provider listed in the Provider box. If she is not, select her name from the Provider drop-down list.

3. Click Monday, February 17 on the calendar.

4. Click Create Break on the Edit menu, or use the Create a Break shortcut button. The break buttons are displayed in the lower left corner of the window.

5. Click the Seminar button.

6. Point to the 8:00 a.m. time-slot box. Press and hold down the left-mouse button and drag to fill all the time slots for February 17. The word "Seminar" is now displayed in all the time slots for February 17. (If any slots are missed, click them to fill them with the seminar break.)

7. Repeat the process for February 18 and 19.

8. Click the Close button at the bottom of the list of break buttons.

**Recurring Breaks
shortcut button.**

RECURRING BREAKS COMMAND

To create recurring breaks, click Recurring Breaks on the Office Hours Edit menu or click the Recurring Breaks shortcut button on the toolbar. The Recurring Breaks dialog box is displayed (see Figure 8-15). There are four tabs in the Recurring Breaks dialog box: Once a Year; Once a Month; Day of Week or Month; and X # of Days, Weeks, or Months.

Once a Year Tab

The Once a Year tab is used to enter a recurring break that occurs once a year (see Figure 8-16). The tab includes the following boxes:

Breaks   The Breaks box lists breaks that have already been created. When a new break is created, it is listed in this box.

Description   The Description box is used to indicate the type of activity, such as a coffee break or business meeting.

Type of Break   In the Type of Break box, the category is selected from a drop-down list.

Start Time   The starting time of the break is entered in the Start Time box, using the counter buttons to move forward or backward.

Length (in minutes)   The duration of the break is entered in the Length (in minutes) box, using the counter buttons to add or delete time in 15-minute increments.

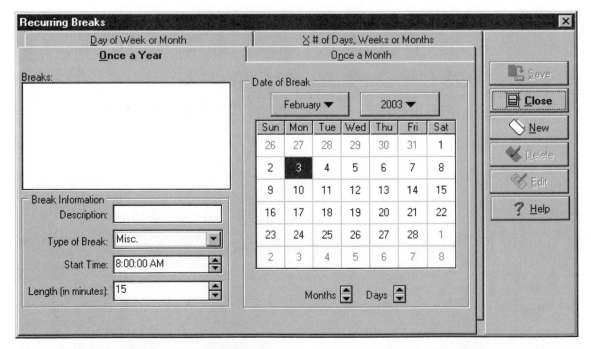

Figure 8-15 Recurring Breaks dialog box.

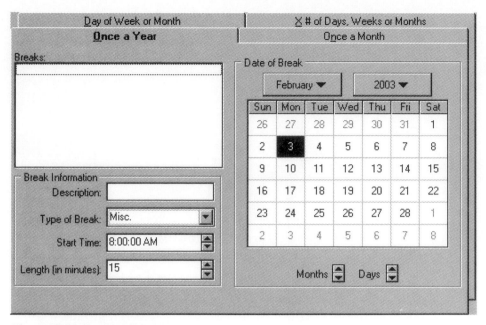

Figure 8-16 Once a Year tab.

Date of Break   The date of the break is selected using drop-down lists for the month and year. The day of the month is entered by clicking the day on the calendar or by using the Days counter buttons to move ahead or back.

The Save button is clicked to save the break information. After the break is saved, it is listed in the Breaks box at the top left of the Once a Year tab.

Once a Month Tab

The Once a Month tab contains the same boxes as the Once a Year tab (see Figure 8-17 on page 168). The Save button is clicked to save the break information. After the break is saved, it is listed in the Breaks box at the top left of the Once a Month tab.

Day of Week or Month Tab

The Day of Week or Month tab is used to enter a recurring break that occurs on a specific day of a week or month (see Figure 8-18 on page 168). For example, a physician's seminar may be held on the first Monday of every month. This tab includes the same boxes as the Once a Year tab and the following additional boxes:

Start Date   The date that the break begins (the first time the break occurs) is entered in the Start Date box.

Day of Week   The day of the week on which the break occurs is entered in the Day of Week box by clicking the corresponding radio

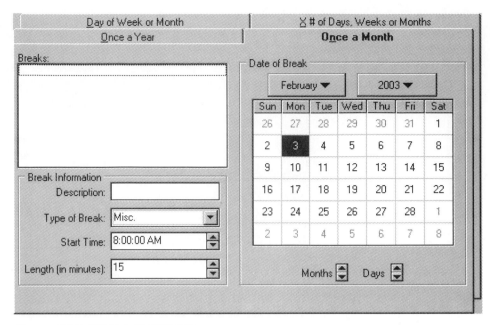

Figure 8-17 Once a Month tab.

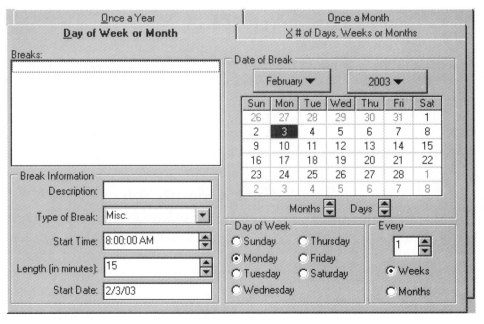

Figure 8-18 Day of Week or Month tab.

button. The day selected in the Day of Week box must be the same day of the week that is highlighted in the calendar.

Every The Every box lists how often the break recurs, either a specified number of weeks or a specified number of months.

The Save button is clicked to save the break information. After the break is saved, it is listed in the Breaks box at the top left of the Day of Week or Month tab.

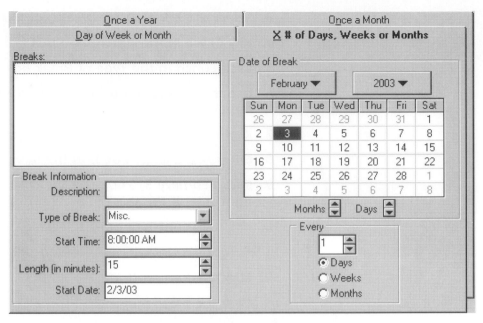

Figure 8-19 X # of Days, Weeks or Months tab.

X # of Days, Weeks or Months Tab

The X # of Days, Weeks or Months tab is used to enter a break that recurs a specified number of days, weeks, or months (see Figure 8-19). For example, a staff meeting is scheduled every day at 8 a.m., or a provider meeting is scheduled every two weeks. This tab includes all the boxes on the Once a Year tab and the following additional boxes:

Start Date The date that the break begins (the first time the break occurs) is entered in the Start Date box.

Every The Every box lists how often the break recurs, a specified number of days, weeks, or months.

The Save button is clicked to save the break information. After the break is saved, it is listed in the Breaks box at the top left of the X # of Days, Weeks or Months tab.

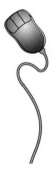

Exercise 8-12

Dr. Katherine Yan takes lunch from 12:00 p.m. to 1:00 p.m. Enter her lunch as a recurring break.

Windows System Date: February 3, 2003

1. **Check that Katherine Yan is the provider listed in the Provider box. If she is not, click her name on the drop-down list.**

2. **Click Recurring Breaks from the Edit menu.**

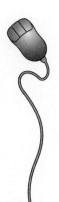

3. Select the X # of Days, Weeks, or Months tab.

4. Key *Lunch* in the Description box.

5. Click Lunch in the Type of Break box.

6. Use the counter buttons to select 12:00 PM in the Start Time box.

7. Key *60* in the Length (in minutes) box.

8. Enter February 3, 2003, in the Start Date box.

9. Click February 3, 2003, on the calendar that appears on the right side of the tab.

10. Use the counter buttons to select 1 in the Every box.

11. Accept the default radio button selection, "days."

12. Click the Save button.

13. Click the Close button.

14. Check to see that the break has been entered on the Office Hours schedule.

PREVIEWING AND PRINTING SCHEDULES

In most medical offices, providers' schedules are printed on a daily basis. To preview a schedule, click Preview Appointment List from the File menu. The appointment list is displayed in a preview window (see Figure 8-20). Various buttons are used to view the schedule at different sizes, to move from page to page, to print the schedule, and to save the schedule as a file. Clicking the Exit button closes the preview window.

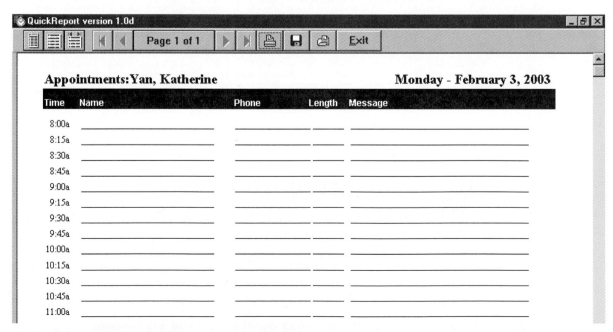

Figure 8-20 Preview window.

Print button.

To print the schedule from within the preview window, the Print button is clicked. The schedule can also be printed directly from the File menu, without using the Preview option. To print from the File menu, click Print Appointment List. The schedule is sent to the printer. (Office Hours prints the schedule for the provider who is listed in the Provider box. To print the schedule of a different provider, change the entry in the Provider box before printing the schedule.)

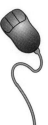

Exercise 8-13

Print Dr. John Rudner's schedule for Monday, February 10, 2003.

Windows System Date: February 3, 2003

1. Select Dr. John Rudner as the provider, if he is not already selected.

2. Go to Monday, February 10, 2003, on the calendar.

3. Click Print Appointment List on the Office Hours File menu, or click the Print Report shortcut button.

4. Check the settings in the Print dialog box, and then click the OK button to print.

5. Close Office Hours.

6. Exit MediSoft.

CHAPTER REVIEW

USING TERMINOLOGY

Define the terms below as they apply to Office Hours.

1. Office Hours schedule

   _____

   _____

2. Office Hours break

   _____

   _____

CHECKING YOUR UNDERSTANDING

Answer the questions below in the space provided.

3. What are the different ways of starting Office Hours?

   _____

   _____

4. How do you display the schedule for the current date for one of the providers in a practice?

   _____

   _____

5. If the calendar shows October 6, how do you move to November 6?

   _____

   _____

6. What MediSoft feature is used to enter breaks that affect all providers and occur on a regular schedule, such as a staff meeting?

   _____

   _____

7. How is an appointment deleted?

   _____

   _____

8. What two menu commands are used to move an appointment from one time slot to another?

_____

_____

9. Suppose your office has set up Office Hours so that the default appointment length is 15 minutes. If you need to make a one-hour appointment for a patient, in what box do you change 15 to 60?

_____

_____

APPLYING KNOWLEDGE

10. After you entered a personal break for Dr. Katherine Yan on February 24, she tells you she gave you the wrong date. The break should be February 25. How do you correct the schedule?

_____

_____

11. A patient calls to request an appointment on a specific day next week. You determine that the appointment is for a routine checkup, not an emergency. What steps should you follow to schedule the appointment?

_____

_____

AT THE COMPUTER

Answer the following questions at the computer:

12. Dr. Katherine Yan asks you to find out when Sarah Fitzwilliams is coming in for her next appointment. Locate the appointment in Office Hours.

13. Today is February 3, 2003. Samuel Bell needs to be scheduled as soon as possible for a 30-minute appointment with Dr. John Rudner, between 2:00 p.m. and 4:00 p.m. Schedule the appointment.

14. Using the List Only feature, display only those patients on the recall list whose status is Call.

15. Set a break for Dr. John Rudner. He will be out of the office March 3, 2003 from 8:00 a.m. until 10:15 a.m.

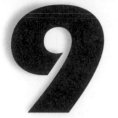

CHAPTER

9

Using Claim Management

WHAT YOU NEED TO KNOW

To use this chapter, you need to know how to:

◆ Start MediSoft, use menus, and enter and edit text.

◆ Work with chart numbers and codes.

OBJECTIVES

In this chapter, you will learn how to:

◆ Create electronic claims.

◆ Review claims for errors and omissions.

◆ Review an audit/edit report.

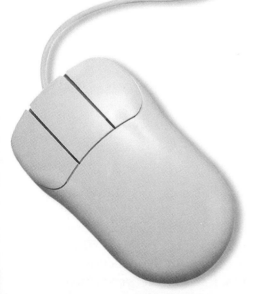

KEY TERMS

filter
navigator buttons

CREATING CLAIMS

Claim Management shortcut button.

Within the Claim Management area of MediSoft, insurance claims are created, edited, and submitted for payment. Claims are created from transactions previously entered in MediSoft. After claims are created, they can either be printed and mailed or transmitted electronically. The Claim Management dialog box is displayed by clicking Claim Management on the Activities menu or by clicking the Claim Management shortcut button on the toolbar (see Figure 9-1). This dialog box lists all claims that have already been created. In this dialog box, several actions can be performed: existing claims can be reviewed and edited, new claims can be created, the status of existing claims can be changed, and claims can be printed or submitted electronically.

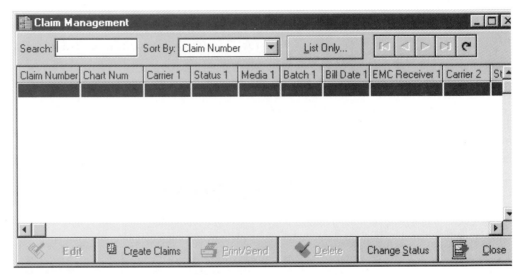

Figure 9-1 Claim Management dialog box.

navigator buttons buttons that simplify the task of moving from one entry to another.

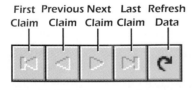

Figure 9-2 Navigator buttons.

The Claim Management dialog box contains five **navigator buttons** that simplify the task of moving from one entry to another (see Figure 9-2). The First Claim button selects the first claim in the list and makes it active. The Previous Claim button reactivates the claim that was most recently active. The Next Claim button makes the next claim in the list active. The Last Claim button makes the last claim in the list active. The Refresh Data button is used to restore data when necessary.

CREATE CLAIMS DIALOG BOX

filter a condition that data must meet to be included in the selection.

Claims are created in the Create Claims dialog box. The Create Claims dialog box (see Figure 9-3) is accessed by clicking the Create Claims button in the Claim Management dialog box. This dialog box provides several filters to customize the creation of claims. A **filter** is a condition that data must meet to be included in the selection of data. For example, claims can be created for services performed

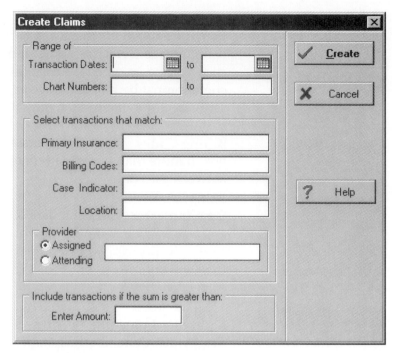

Figure 9-3 Create Claims dialog box.

between the first and the fifteenth of the month. If this were the case, the filter would be the condition that services must have been performed between the first and fifteenth of the month. Transactions that meet this criteria would be included in the selection; transactions that do not fall within that date range are not included. Filters can be used to create claims for a specific patient, for a specific insurance carrier, for transactions that exceed a certain dollar amount, and others. The following filters can be applied within the Create Claims dialog box.

Range of The options in this section of the dialog box provide filters for establishing the starting and ending dates as well as the starting and ending chart numbers for the claims that will be created.

Transaction Dates The Transaction Dates boxes are used to specify the starting and ending dates for which claims will be created. If the boxes are left blank, transactions for all dates will be included.

Chart Numbers In the Chart Numbers boxes, the starting and ending chart numbers for which claims will be created are entered. If the boxes are left blank, all chart numbers will be included.

Select Transactions That Match The options in this section of the dialog box provide filters for matching the exact primary insurance carrier(s), billing code(s), case indicator(s), and location(s).

Primary Insurance The carrier code for the insurance company is entered in the Primary Insurance box. If claims are being sent to a clearinghouse, more than one insurance carrier code can be entered. When more than one code is entered, a comma must be placed between the codes. If claims are being sent directly to the carrier, only that carrier's code is entered.

Billing Codes The billing code is entered in the Billing Codes box. If more than one code is entered, a comma must be placed between the codes.

Case Indicator If case indicators are used to classify patients (such as by type of illness for workers' compensation cases), the case indicator can be listed in the Case Indicator box. If more than one indicator is entered, a comma must be placed between each one.

Location Sometimes a sort is needed by location, such as all procedures done at a hospital. The location code is entered in the Location box. If more than one code is entered, a comma must be placed between the codes.

Provider The radio buttons in the Provider box indicate whether the provider is the assigned or attending provider. In the box to the right of the radio buttons, the provider code is entered. If more than one code is entered, a comma must be placed between the codes.

Include Transactions if the Sum Is Greater Than The dollar amount entered in this box is the minimum total amount required for a case before a claim can be created.

Any box that is not filled in will default to include all data, and claims with any entry in that box will be included. When all necessary information has been entered, clicking the Create button creates the claims. MediSoft will create a file of matching claims but will only include those that have not yet been billed.

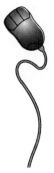

Exercise 9-1

Create insurance claims for all patients who have transactions not already placed on a claim. (The program uses the Windows System Date when creating claims. Be sure to set not only the MediSoft Program Date but also the Windows System Date before beginning the exercises in this chapter.)

MediSoft Program Date: January 30, 2004

Windows System Date: January 30, 2004

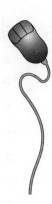

1. **Start MediSoft.**

2. **On the Activities menu, click Claim Management. The Claim Management dialog box is displayed.**

3. **Click the Create Claims button.**

4. **Leave all boxes blank to select all transactions.**

5. **Click the Create button.**

6. **Use the scroll bars to view the claims just created.**

7. **Click the Close button.**

CLAIM SELECTION

At times it is necessary to select and view specific claims that have already been created. For example, any claims prepared for submission to an insurance carrier must be selected and then reviewed for completeness and accuracy. In addition, all claims that have been rejected by insurance carriers are selected and reviewed before resubmission.

MediSoft's List Only feature is used when it is necessary to list claims that match certain criteria. Filters are applied in the List Only Claims That Match dialog box. They can be used to view claims selectively, for example, claims for a specific insurance carrier, claims created on a certain date, and so on. Unlike the filters in the Create Claims dialog box, those in the List Only Claims That Match dialog box do not create claims; they simply list existing claims that meet the specified criteria.

Once the filters have been applied, only those claims that match the criteria are listed at the bottom of the main Claim Management dialog box. Claims can be sorted by chart number, date the claim was created, insurance carrier, electronic media claim (EMC) receiver, billing method, billing date, batch number, and claim status. Not all the boxes need to be filled in, only the ones that will be used to select the desired claims.

The List Only feature is activated by clicking the List Only... button in the Claim Management dialog box. This causes the List Only Claims That Match dialog box to display (see Figure 9-4 on page 180).

The following filters are available in the List Only Claims That Match dialog box:

Chart Number   A patient's chart number is selected from the drop-down list of patients' chart numbers.

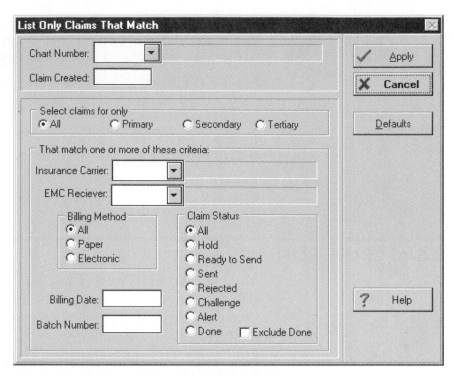

Figure 9-4 List Only Claims That Match dialog box.

Claim Created   The date that a claim was created is entered in MMDDYY format.

Select Claims for Only   A radio button is clicked for either all insurance carriers, primary insurance carrier only, secondary insurance carrier only, or tertiary insurance carrier only. When a patient has insurance coverage with more than one carrier, the primary carrier is billed first, and then, if appropriate, the second and third (tertiary) carriers are billed.

Insurance Carrier   An insurance carrier is selected from the drop-down list of choices.

EMC Receiver   An EMC receiver is selected from the choices on the drop-down list.

Billing Method   In the Billing Method box, the radio button for All, Paper, or Electronic is clicked.

Billing Date   The date of billing is entered in the Billing Date box.

Batch Number   A batch number is entered in the Batch Number box.

Claim Status   A claim status is selected from the list of radio buttons provided. If claims that have been billed and accepted (not rejected) are to be excluded from the search, the Exclude Done box is clicked. This causes a check mark to display beside the option.

When the desired boxes have been filled in, clicking the Apply button applies the selected filters to the claims data. The Claim Management dialog box is displayed listing only those claims that match the criteria selected in the List Only Claims That Match dialog box. From the Claim Management dialog box, the claims can now be edited, printed and mailed, or transmitted electronically. To restore the List Only Claims That Match dialog box to its original settings (that is, to unapply the filters selected), this dialog box is reopened, the Defaults button is clicked, and then the Apply button is clicked. All of the boxes in the dialog box will become blank, and the full list of claims is displayed again in the Claim Management dialog box.

EDITING CLAIMS

MediSoft's Claim Edit feature allows claims to be reviewed and verified on screen before they are submitted to insurance carriers for payment. With careful checking, problems can be solved before claims are sent to insurance carriers. When a claim is active in the Claim Management dialog box, it can be edited by clicking the Edit button or by double-clicking the claim itself. The Claim dialog box is displayed (see Figure 9-5). The top section of the Claim dialog box lists the claim number, the date the claim was created, the chart number, the patient's name, and the case number. This information cannot be edited, although the information in the five tabs can be edited.

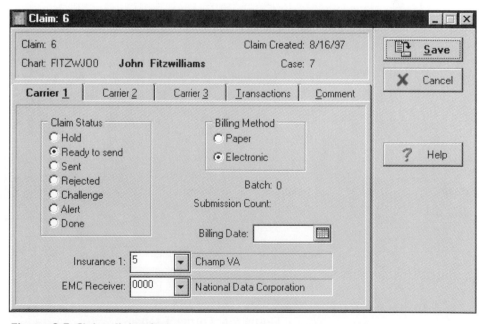

Figure 9-5 Claim dialog box.

CARRIER 1 TAB The Carrier 1 tab displays information about claims being submitted to a patient's primary insurance carrier (see Figure 9-6).

The following boxes are listed in the Carrier 1 tab:

Claim Status The Claim Status box indicates the status of a particular claim: Hold, Ready to send, Sent, Rejected, Challenge, Alert, and Done. The radio button that reflects a claim's status should be clicked.

Billing Method The Billing Method box displays two choices: Paper or Electronic. The radio button that describes the billing method should be clicked.

Batch If the claim has been assigned to a batch, the batch number is displayed.

Submission Count The Submission Count area lists the number of claims submitted.

Billing Date The Billing Date box lists the date the bill was sent.

Insurance 1 The Insurance 1 box lists a patient's primary insurance carrier.

EMC Receiver The EMC receiver is selected from the drop-down list.

CARRIER 2 AND CARRIER 3 TABS The Carrier 2 and Carrier 3 tabs display information about claims being submitted to a patient's secondary (Carrier 2) and tertiary (Carrier 3) insurance carriers. The boxes in these tabs are the same as the boxes in the Carrier 1 tab.

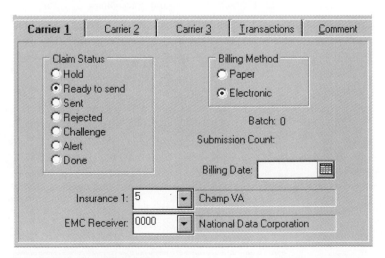

Figure 9-6 Carrier 1 tab.

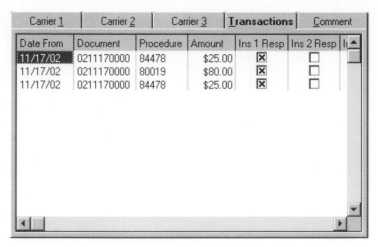

Figure 9-7 Transactions tab.

TRANSACTIONS TAB

The Transactions tab lists information about the transactions included in a claim. The scroll bars can be used to view all the information in the Transactions tab (see Figure 9-7).

Date From The Date From box lists the date service was provided.

Document The Document box lists the document number of a transaction.

Procedure The Procedure box displays the procedure code for a procedure performed.

Amount In the Amount box, the dollar cost of a service is displayed.

Ins 1 Resp If this box has an "X" in it, the primary insurance carrier is responsible for the claim.

Ins 2 Resp If this box has an "X" in it, the secondary insurance carrier is responsible for the claim.

Ins 3 Resp If this box has an "X" in it, the tertiary insurance carrier is responsible for the claim.

COMMENT TAB

The Comment tab provides a place to include any specific notes or comments about the claim (see Figure 9-8 on page 184).

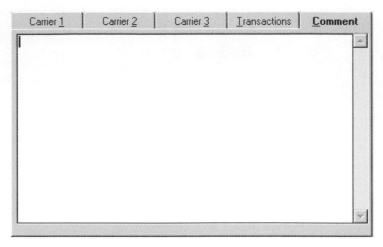

| Carrier 1 | Carrier 2 | Carrier 3 | Transactions | **Comment** |

Figure 9-8 Comment tab.

Exercise 9-2

Perform a search to locate the code for East Ohio PPO. Review insurance claims for patients with East Ohio PPO as their insurance carrier.

MediSoft Program Date: January 30, 2004

Windows System Date: January 30, 2004

1. Click Insurance Carriers on the Lists menu.

2. Begin the search for East Ohio PPO by clicking Name in the Sort By box.

3. In the Search box, key *East*. Notice that the selection arrow now points to the entry for East Ohio PPO and that the code for East Ohio PPO is 13.

4. Close the Insurance Carrier List dialog box.

5. Open the Claim Management dialog box.

6. Click the List Only... button.

7. Click 13 East Ohio PPO on the drop-down list in the Insurance Carrier box.

8. Click the Apply button. You are returned to the Claim Management dialog box. Notice that only claims for patients who have East Ohio PPO as their insurance carrier are listed.

9. Double-click Chart Number BELLSARØ or click the Edit button to review the claim for Sarina Bell. The Claim dialog box is displayed.

10. Review the information in the Carrier 1 tab.

11. Review the information in the Transactions tab.

12. Click the Cancel button to exit the Claim dialog box without saving any changes. (The Cancel button does not cancel the claim; it just cancels any changes that may have been made in the Claim dialog box.)

ELECTRONIC MEDIA CLAIMS

Many of the setup and entry requirements for electronic media claims (EMC) are typically handled by the medical office's systems manager. Insurance carriers and clearinghouses that receive claims electronically have different requirements regarding what information needs to be included on an electronic claim. Each insurance carrier has specific data requirements, indicating which boxes are mandatory and what the data format should be. The office systems manager maintains detailed information on the EMC requirements of each carrier and updates this information as necessary. However, some basic steps that need to be followed to submit electronic claims are common to most insurance carriers.

STEPS IN SUBMITTING ELECTRONIC CLAIMS

There are a number of steps in the process of submitting electronic claims.

1. Enter information on a patient in the usual manner.
2. Check to make sure all the information required by an insurance carrier is complete; otherwise, the claim will be rejected.
3. Enter transactions and payments as usual.
4. Create claims either through the Transaction Entry dialog box or through the Claim Management feature.
5. Review claims through the Claims Edit and the List Only features to locate any obvious errors.
6. Transmit claims to the clearinghouse.
7. Review the audit/edit report that arrives from the clearinghouse. The audit/edit report lists any problems with the claims. Correct and resubmit any claims that had errors.
8. The clearinghouse transmits the claims to an insurance carrier. The information is received by the insurance carrier and stored in its database, awaiting processing.

TRANSMITTING ELECTRONIC CLAIMS IN MEDISOFT

After making sure all the information is complete and correct for claims being sent, the Print/Send button in the Claim Management dialog box is clicked. This causes the Print/Send Claims dialog box to display. Within this dialog box, the billing method (paper or electronic) must be indicated (see Figure 9-9 on page 186). If the claims being sent are paper, the Paper radio button is clicked. If the claims are being submitted electronically, the Electronic radio button is clicked.

When the Electronic radio button is clicked, the Electronic Claim Receiver box becomes active. The EMC receiver is selected from the list of choices in the drop-down list. After the EMC receiver has been selected and the OK button is clicked, the Send Electronic Claims dialog box is displayed (see Figure 9-10 on page 186). This dialog

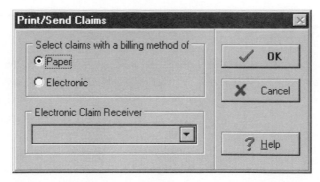

Figure 9-9 Print/Send Claims dialog box.

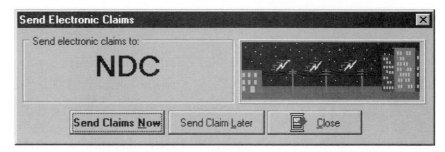

Figure 9-10 Send Electronic Claims dialog box.

box provides the option of sending claims now or sending claims later, via the Send Claims Now and Send Claims Later buttons. After claims are sent, the system marks them "Sent."

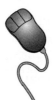

Exercise 9-3

Prepare to send electronic claims to a clearinghouse.

MediSoft Program Date: January 30, 2004

Windows System Date: January 30, 2004

1. In the Claim Management dialog box, click the Print/Send button.

2. In the Print/Send Claims dialog box, select claims with an electronic billing method by clicking the Electronic radio button.

3. Click National Data Corporation on the drop-down list in the Electronic Claim Receiver box.

4. Click the OK button. The Send Electronic Claims dialog box is displayed.

5. If you were in a medical office and ready to send claims, you would click the Send Claims Now button. However, because you are in a school setting and are not actually set up to submit electronic claims, click the Close button.

6. Close the Claim Management dialog box.

```
█VENDOR TEST PROV          NDC CLAIMS AUDIT/EDIT REPORT  08/05/97  5:27PM PAGE    1
█* TEST - NO DATA FORWARDED *         MEDICAL    (5.0)              STATION : 001
█ PAT ACCT#    CLM# PATIENT NAME       MESSAGE                          AMOUNT FLG
█JETGE000      00001 JETSON,G   **>MISSING LINE ITEM CHARGE            LINE  1  R
JETGE000       00001 JETSON,G   **>MISSING PATIENT MEDICARE NUMBER             R


ROARU000       00002 ROAD,R     **>MISSING MEDICARE NUMBER SUFFIX              R

COYWI000       00003 COYOTE,W      CLAIM WILL BE FORWARDED TO AETNA   $  65.00
█VENDOR TEST PROV          ETS CLAIMS AUDIT/EDIT REPORT  08/05/97  5:27PM LAST PAGE
█* TEST - NO DATA FORWARDED *         MEDICAL    (5.0)              STATION : 001
█  CARRIER     CLMS-RCV   AMT-RCV     CLMS-FWD   AMT-FWD    CLMS-REJ   AMT-REJ
█COMM. INS        1        65.00         1        65.00        0         0.00
MEDICARE          2        65.00         0         0.00        2        65.00
               ----  ------------     ----  ------------    ----  ------------
GRAND TOTAL       3       130.00         1        65.00        2        65.00
                                                                  *            *
                                                                  *            *
****************************************************************************
*  THIS AMT. WOULD HAVE BEEN PENDED,SUSPENDED OR REJECTED BY INSURANCE CARRIER *
****************************************************************************
█                                                                ACCEPTED  33%
█*TEST*TEST*TEST*TEST*TEST*TEST*TEST*TEST*TEST*TEST*TEST*TEST*TEST*TEST*TEST*TEST
█
█
```

Figure 9-11 Audit/Edit report.

REVIEWING THE AUDIT/EDIT REPORT

When claims are transmitted to a clearinghouse, an audit/edit report is received from it immediately after claims are sent (see Figure 9-11). Options for viewing the report are listed on-screen when the report is received. The audit/edit report marks each claim as accepted or rejected.

Each claim is displayed on a separate line of the report. The Message column queries whether a claim will be sent to an insurance carrier. If a claim cannot be sent, the error is listed in the Message column. In the Flag column of the report, a "P" indicates that the claim will be sent on paper; an "R" indicates the claim was rejected. A blank Flag column means that the claim will be sent electronically. The report should be reviewed carefully. Any errors found by a clearinghouse must be corrected before a claim can be sent to an insurance carrier.

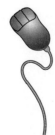

Exercise 9-4

An audit/edit report has come back from the clearinghouse. A claim for James Smith has been rejected for submission to Blue Cross/Blue Shield. There are two reasons listed for rejection: "Missing Insured's ID no." and "Missing Insured's Group no.". Locate the problem in MediSoft, correct it, and prepare the claim for resubmission.

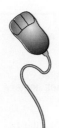

MediSoft Program Date: January 30, 2004

Windows System Date: January 30, 2004

1. Go to the Policy 1 tab in the Case dialog box to check whether Mr. Smith's insurance policy number and group number have been entered.

2. Notice that these boxes are blank. Someone forgot to enter data in them when creating the case for Mr. Smith.

3. Key *354691* in the Policy Number box.

4. Key *U339* in the Group Number box.

5. Click the Save button.

6. Close the Patient List dialog box.

7. Double-click the rejected claim in the Claim Management dialog box to edit the claim.

8. Change the claim status from Rejected to Ready to Send. Click the Save button.

9. Close the Claim Management dialog box. (In an actual office setting, the claim would now be resent to the clearinghouse. Because schools are not set up to transmit electronic media claims, this exercise ends with Step 10.)

10. Exit MediSoft.

CHAPTER REVIEW

USING TERMINOLOGY

Define the terms below.

1. filter

_____

_____

2. navigator buttons

_____

_____

CHECKING YOUR UNDERSTANDING

Answer the questions below in the space provided.

3. A claim needs to be submitted for John Fitzwilliams. How would you select only those claims pertaining to John Fitzwilliams?

_____

_____

4. On an audit/edit report, what does an "R" in the Flag column indicate?

_____

_____

5. If an error is found on a claim, how is it corrected?

_____

_____

APPLYING KNOWLEDGE

Answer the questions below in the space provided.

6. You were asked to create claims for Samuel Bell. After entering his chart number in the Create Claims dialog box, you receive the message "No new claims were created." Why were no claims created for Samuel Bell?

_____

_____

CHAPTER REVIEW

_____

_____

AT THE COMPUTER

Answer the following questions at the computer:

7. Locate all claims ready to be submitted to Ohio Central Health Plan.

8. Change the status of James Smolowski's claim from Ready to Send to Hold.

9. Locate all claims that are ready to be submitted for Randall Klein.

10 Printing Reports

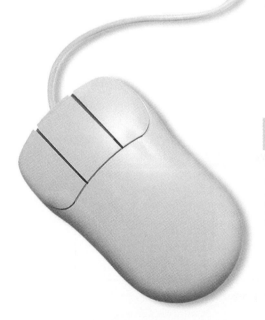

WHAT YOU NEED TO KNOW

To use this chapter, you need to know how to:
- ◆ Start MediSoft, use menus, and enter and edit text.
- ◆ Work with chart numbers and codes.

OBJECTIVES

In this chapter, you will learn how to:
- ◆ Select the options available for different reports.
- ◆ Preview and print a variety of MediSoft reports.
- ◆ Access MediSoft's Report Designer.

KEY TERMS

aging report	patient statement
patient day sheet	procedure day sheet
patient ledger	

REPORTS IN THE MEDICAL OFFICE

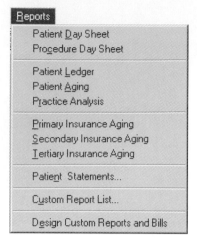

Figure 10-1 Reports menu.

Reports are an important tool in managing a medical office. They provide useful information about a practice and its patients. Providers and office managers ask for different reports at different times. Some providers want to see a daily report of each day's transactions. Others want to see reports on particular patients' accounts on a weekly or bimonthly basis.

MediSoft provides a variety of standard reports, and has the ability to create custom reports using the Report Designer. Standard and custom reports are accessed through the Reports menu (see Figure 10-1). The Reports menu lists standard reports and also provides choices designing custom reports using the Report Designer.

STANDARD REPORTS

The standard reports are patient day sheets, procedure day sheets, patient ledger, patient aging, practice analysis, insurance aging reports, and patient statements.

Patient Day Sheet

patient day sheet *a summary of the activity of patient accounts on any given day.*

At the end of the day, many medical practices print a **patient day sheet**, which is a summary of the activity of patient activity on any given day (see Figures 10-2a and 10-2b). MediSoft's version of this report lists the procedures for a particular day, grouped by patient, in alphabetical order by chart number. It includes:

◆ Procedures performed for a particular patient or group of patients.

◆ Charges, receipts, adjustments, and balances for a particular patient or group of patients.

◆ A summary of a practice's charges, payments, and adjustments.

To print a patient day sheet, Patient Day Sheet is clicked on the Reports menu. The Print Report Where? dialog box is displayed, asking whether the report should be previewed on the screen or sent

---

Family Care Center
Patient Day Sheet
March 3, 2003

Entry	Date	Document	POS	Description	Provider	Code	Amount
KLEINRA0		**Randall Klein**					
47	3/3/03	0303030000	11		2	99212	40.00
48	3/3/03	0303030000	11		2	29425	30.00
49	3/3/03	0303030000	11		2	99070	20.00
		Today's Charges		Today's Receipts	Adjustments		Patient Balance
		$90.00		$0.00	$0.00		$90.00

Figure 10-2a Page 1 of Patient Day Sheet report.

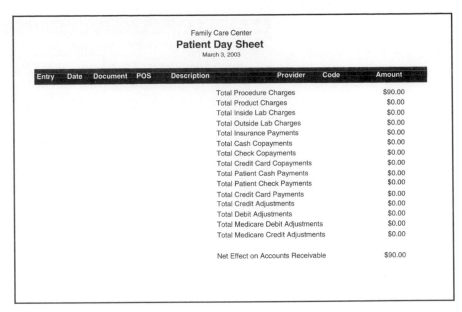

Figure 10-2b Page 2 of Patient Day Sheet report.

directly to the printer (see Figure 10-3). Reports that are previewed on the screen can also be printed from the Preview Report window. When the Preview the Report on the Screen radio button is selected and the Start button is clicked, the Data Selection Questions dialog box is displayed (see Figure 10-4 on page 194). This dialog box provides the opportunity to select the patients, dates, and providers for whom a report is being generated. If any box is left blank, all values are included in the report. For example, if no chart numbers are entered, all patients will be included in the report.

Chart Number Range In the Chart Number Range boxes, a range of chart numbers for patients is entered. If a report is needed for just one patient, that patient's chart number is entered in both boxes.

Date Created Range A range of dates when transactions were entered in MediSoft is entered in the two boxes. The Windows System Date is the default entry. If this is not the date desired, it can be changed by selecting new dates and entering them.

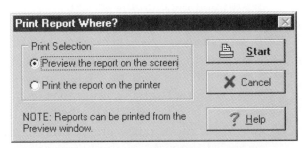

Figure 10-3 Print Report Where? dialog box.

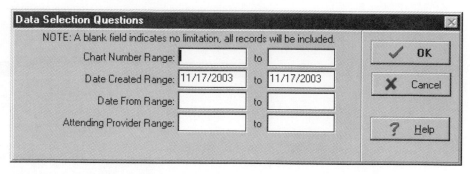

Figure 10-4 Data Selection Questions dialog box.

Date From Range   A range of dates is entered in the Date From Range boxes. For example, if it were necessary to print patient day sheets for the period of May 1 to May 15, 2003, "050103" would be entered in the first box and "051503" in the second box. If transactions were needed for the current date, that date would be entered in both boxes.

Attending Provider Range   A range of codes for the attending providers is entered in the Attending Provider Range boxes.

When these selection boxes have been completed, the OK button is clicked. MediSoft begins creating the report. MediSoft generates the report and displays it on-screen or sends it to the printer, depending on the selection made in the Print Report Where? dialog box.

The Preview Report window, common to all reports, provides options for viewing or printing a report (see Figure 10-5). The buttons on the Preview Report toolbar control how a report is displayed on-screen and how movement is done from page to page within a report (see Figure 10-6).

The three zoom buttons at the left of the toolbar are used to affect the size of the report displayed on-screen. The zoom button farthest to the left reduces a report so that a full page fits on the screen. The middle zoom button displays a report at 100 percent size. This option acts like a magnifying glass, allowing a portion of a report to be viewed up close. The zoom button on the right displays the full width of a page on the screen.

A series of four triangle buttons, two on the left and two on the right, are used to move through pages of a multipage report. The First Page button farthest on the left, moves to the beginning of a report. The Previous Page button moves to the page that precedes the one currently displayed. The bar between the four triangle buttons indicates how many pages are in a report and the number of the current page. To the right of the bar are the other two additional triangle

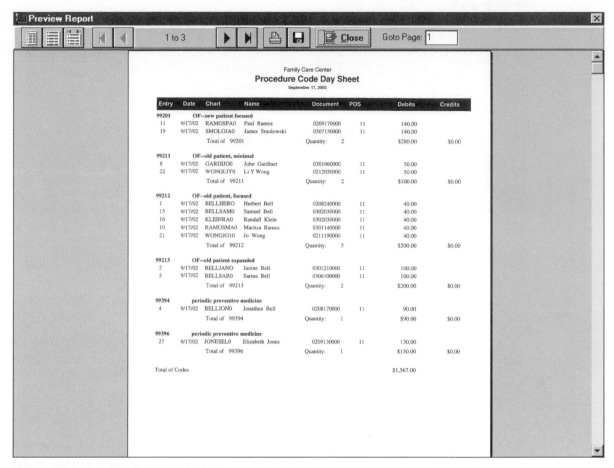

Figure 10-5 Preview Report window.

buttons. The Next Page button moves to the page following the current one. The Last Page button moves to the end of a report.

The remaining buttons include the Print button, which is used to send a report to the printer, and the Disk button, which saves a report to disk. The Close button closes the Preview Report window, redisplaying the main MediSoft window.

The Preview Report window also contains the Go to Page box, in which the number of a specific page to be displayed in the Preview Report window is entered.

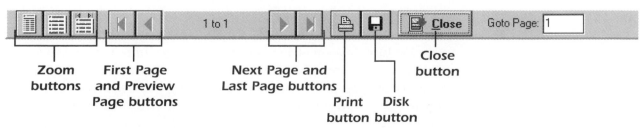

Figure 10-6 Buttons on Preview Report toolbar.

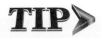

TIP Most of the standard MediSoft reports use the Windows System Date, not the MediSoft Program Date. The Windows System Date is used as the default entry in the Date Created Range boxes. This default entry can be overridden by keying in the desired date(s).

Exercise 10-1

Print a patient day sheet report for March 3, 2003 with the entire range of chart numbers, dates from, and attending providers. (That is, leave all data selection boxes blank.)

MediSoft Program Date: March 3, 2003

Windows System Date: March 3, 2003

1. Start MediSoft.

2. On the Reports menu, click Patient Day Sheet. The Print Report Where? dialog box is displayed.

3. Click the radio button for previewing the report on-screen if it is not already selected. Click the Start button. The Data Selection Questions dialog box is displayed.

4. Accept the default entry of 3/3/2003 in both of the Date Created Range boxes. (If a different date is displayed, change it by keying *03032003*.) Leave all other boxes blank. This will select data for all patients and attending providers for March 3, 2003. Click the OK button. The patient day sheet report is displayed.

5. Click the appropriate zoom button on the toolbar to display the report the full width of the screen so it is easier to read.

6. Scroll down the page to view additional entries on the first page of the report.

7. Click the Next Page button to advance to the second page of the report.

8. Click the other zoom and triangle buttons on the toolbar to see their effects. Use the Go to Page box to move back to page one of the report.

9. Click the Print button to send the report to the printer. Then click the OK button on the Print menu.

10. Click the Close button to exit the Preview Report window.

Procedure Day Sheet

procedure day sheet *a list of all the procedures performed on a particular day.*

A **procedure day sheet** lists all of the procedures performed on a particular day, and gives the dates, patients, document numbers, places of service, debits, and credits relating to these procedures (see Figure 10-7). Procedures are listed in numerical order. Procedure

Family Care Center
Procedure Code Day Sheet
September 17, 2002

Entry	Date	Chart	Name	Document	POS	Debits	Credits
99201		**OF--new patient focused**					
11	9/17/02	RAMOSPA0	Paul Ramos	0209170000	11	140.00	
19	9/17/02	SMOLOJA0	James Smolowski	0307150000	11	140.00	
		Total of 99201		Quantity: 2		$280.00	$0.00
99211		**OF--old patient, minimal**					
8	9/17/02	GARDIJO0	John Gardiner	0301060000	11	50.00	
22	9/17/02	WONGLIY0	Li Y Wong	0212050000	11	50.00	
		Total of 99211		Quantity: 2		$100.00	$0.00
99212		**OF--old patient, focused**					
1	9/17/02	BELLHER0	Herbert Bell	0208240000	11	40.00	
15	9/17/02	BELLSAM0	Samuel Bell	0302030000	11	40.00	
16	9/17/02	KLEINRA0	Randall Klein	0302030000	11	40.00	
10	9/17/02	RAMOSMA0	Maritza Ramos	0301140000	11	40.00	
21	9/17/02	WONGJO10	Jo Wong	0211190000	11	40.00	
		Total of 99212		Quantity: 5		$200.00	$0.00
99213		**OF--old patient expanded**					
2	9/17/02	BELLJAN0	Janine Bell	0301210000	11	100.00	
5	9/17/02	BELLSAR0	Sarina Bell	0306100000	11	100.00	
		Total of 99213		Quantity: 2		$200.00	$0.00
99394		**periodic preventive medicine**					
4	9/17/02	BELLJON0	Jonathan Bell	0208170000	11	90.00	
		Total of 99394		Quantity: 1		$90.00	$0.00
99396		**periodic preventive medicine**					
27	9/17/02	JONESEL0	Elizabeth Jones	0209130000	11	130.00	
		Total of 99396		Quantity: 1		$130.00	$0.00
Total of Codes						$1,567.00	

Figure 10-7 Procedure Day Sheet report.

day sheets are printed by clicking Procedure Day Sheet on the Reports menu. The same Print Report Where? dialog box used for a patient day sheet is displayed. Again, the report can be previewed on-screen or printed directly.

Once the decision to preview or print is made, the data selection criteria must be determined. The Data Selection Questions dialog box provides options to select by procedure codes, dates, and providers (see Figure 10-8 on page 198). A procedure day sheet will be generated only for the data that meets the selection criteria. If any box is left blank, all values are included in the report.

The following boxes are listed in the Data Selection Questions dialog box:

Code 1 Range   In the Code 1 Range box, a range of procedure codes is entered. If a report is needed for a single code, it is entered in both boxes.

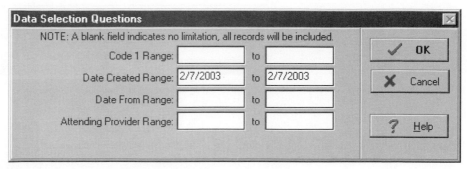

Data Selection Questions

NOTE: A blank field indicates no limitation, all records will be included.

Code 1 Range:		to	
Date Created Range:	2/7/2003	to	2/7/2003
Date From Range:		to	
Attending Provider Range:		to	

✓ OK
✗ Cancel
? Help

Figure 10-8 Data Selection Questions dialog box.

Date Created Range A range of dates when transactions were entered in MediSoft is entered in the two boxes. The Windows system date is the default entry. If this is not the date desired, it can be changed by selecting new dates and entering them.

Date From Range A range of dates when each transaction occurred is entered in the Date From Range boxes.

Attending Provider Range Codes for attending providers are entered in the Attending Provider Range boxes.

Exercise 10-2

Print a procedure day sheet report for March 3, 2003 with the entire range of procedure codes, dates from, and attending providers.

MediSoft Program Date: March 3, 2003

Windows System Date: March 3, 2003

1. On the Reports menu, click Procedure Day Sheet. The Print Report Where? dialog box is displayed.

2. Click the radio button option for previewing the report on-screen. Click the Start button. The Data Selection Questions dialog box is displayed.

3. Notice that 3/3/2003 is already listed in both Date Created Range boxes. Leave the other boxes blank. Click the OK button. The procedure day sheet report is displayed.

4. View the report at the full width of the screen.

5. Send the report to the printer.

6. Exit the Preview Report window.

Patient Ledger

A **patient ledger** lists the financial activity in each patient's account, including charges, payments, and adjustments (see Figure 10-9). This information is especially useful if there is a question about a patient's account. A full set of patient ledgers details the status of every patient's account.

Patient ledgers are printed by clicking Patient Ledger on the Reports menu. The Print Report Where? dialog box is displayed. After the preview or print selection is made, the Data Selection Questions dialog box is displayed as it is with the other reports (see Figure 10-10). It provides options to select by chart numbers, patient reference balances, dates, and providers. A patient ledger is generated only for data that meet the selection criteria. If any selection box is left blank, all values are included in the report.

Chart Number Range   In the Chart Number Range box, a range of chart numbers for patients is entered. If a report is needed for just one patient, that patient's chart number is entered in both boxes.

Patient Reference Balance Range   Minimum and maximum dollar amounts are entered in the Patient Reference Balance Range boxes to

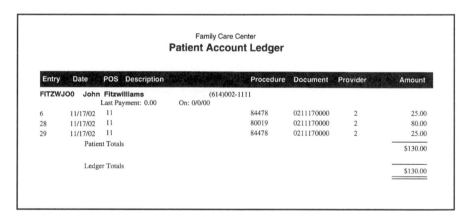

Figure 10-9 Patient Ledger report.

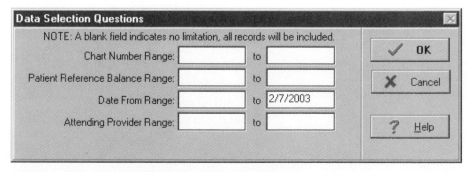

Figure 10-10 Data Selection Questions dialog box.

delineate the dollar amount of an outstanding balance. The amounts are entered with decimal points.

Date From Range   A range of dates is entered in the Date From Range boxes. The system uses the Windows system date as the default entry in the second of these two boxes. If this is not the desired end date, enter the correct one.

Attending Provider Range   Codes for attending providers are entered in the Attending Provider Range boxes.

Exercise 10-3

Print patient ledgers for August 2002 for patients whose last names begin with the letters "A" through "K."

MediSoft Program Date: August 31, 2002

Windows System Date: August 31, 2002

1. On the Reports menu, click Patient Ledger.

2. If necessary, click the radio button for previewing the report on-screen. Click the Start button.

3. Key *A* in the first box of the Chart Number Range box and *K* in the second.

4. Accept the default entries in the Patient Reference Balance Range boxes.

5. In the first box of the Date From Range boxes, enter August 1, 2002 in MMDDCCYY format. Accept the default entry in the second of the boxes.

6. Leave the Attending Provider Range boxes blank.

7. Click the OK button.

8. View the report at the full width of the screen.

9. Send the report to the printer.

10. Exit the Preview Report window.

Patient Aging Report

aging report a report listing the amount of money owed, organized by the amount of time the money has been owed.

An **aging report** lists the amount of money owed, organized by the amount of time the money has been owed. A patient aging report lists a patient's balance by age, the date of the last payment, and the telephone number. The columns display the amounts that are current and those that are 31–60, 61–90, and more than 90 days past due (see Figure 10-11). The aging begins on the date of the transaction.

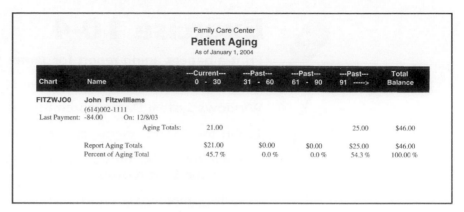

Chart	Name	---Current--- 0 - 30	---Past--- 31 - 60	---Past--- 61 - 90	---Past--- 91 ---->	Total Balance

Family Care Center
Patient Aging
As of January 1, 2004

FITZWJO0 John Fitzwilliams
(614)002-1111
Last Payment: -84.00   On: 12/8/03
Aging Totals: 21.00   25.00 $46.00

Report Aging Totals $21.00 $0.00 $0.00 $25.00 $46.00
Percent of Aging Total   45.7 %   0.0 %   0.0 %   54.3 %   100.00 %

Figure 10-11 Patient Aging report.

Patient aging reports are printed by clicking Patient Aging on the Reports menu. After making a selection in the Print Report Where? dialog box, the data must be selected. The boxes in the Data Selection Questions dialog box are as follows (See Figure 10-12):

Chart Number Range   In the Chart Number Range boxes, a range of chart numbers for patients is entered. If the report is needed for just one patient, that patient's chart number is entered in both boxes.

Date From Range   A range of dates is entered in the Date From Range boxes. The system enters the Windows system date as the default entry in the second of these two boxes.

Attending Provider Range   Codes for attending providers are entered in the Attending Provider Range boxes.

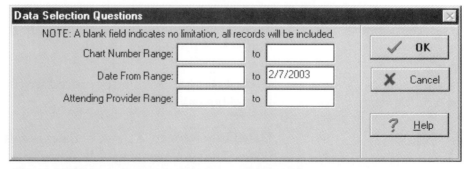

Figure 10-12 Data Selection Questions dialog box.

Exercise 10-4

Print a patient aging report for James Smolowski.

MediSoft Program Date: September 30, 2003

Windows System Date: September 30, 2003

1. On the Reports menu, click Patient Aging.

2. Click the radio button for previewing the report on-screen. Click the Start button.

3. Enter Smolowski's chart number in both boxes of the Chart Number Range boxes. (If you do not remember his chart number, go to the Patient List dialog box and enter the first three letters of his last name in the Search box.)

4. Leave the starting date in the first of the Date From Range boxes blank, and accept the default entry of "9/30/2003" in the second of the boxes.

5. Leave the Attending Provider Range boxes blank. Click the OK button.

6. View the report on-screen.

7. Print the report.

8. Exit the Preview Report window.

Practice Analysis Report

MediSoft's practice analysis report analyzes the revenue of a practice for a specified period of time, usually a month or a year (see Figures 10-13a and 10-13b). The report can be used to generate medical practice financial statements. It can also be used for profit analysis. The summary at the end of the report breaks down the report into total charges, total lab charges (both inside and outside), total patient payments, co-payments, credit card payments, insurance payments, and total credits and debits by both patient and insurance. The following boxes are listed in the Data Selection Questions dialog box (see Figure 10-14):

Code 1 Range   A range of procedure codes is entered in the Code 1 Range boxes.

Date From Range   A range of dates is entered in the Date From Range boxes. The system enters the Windows System Date as the default entry in the second of the two boxes. To change this date, highlight the default entry and enter the new date in MMDDCCYY format.

Attending Provider Range   Codes for attending providers are entered in the Attending Provider Range boxes.

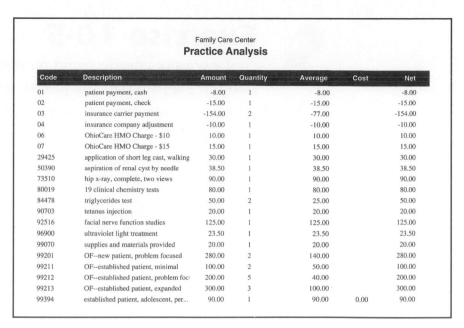

Figure 10-13a Page 1 of Practice Analysis report.

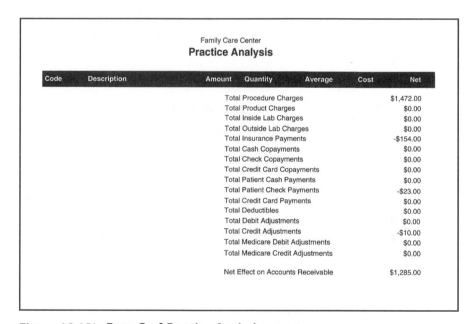

Figure 10-13b Page 2 of Practice Analysis report.

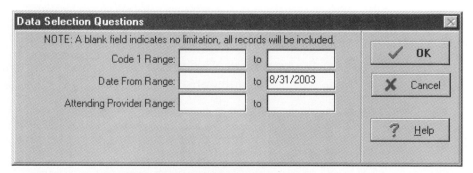

Figure 10-14 Data Selection Questions dialog box.

Exercise 10-5

Print a practice analysis report for August 2002.

MediSoft Program Date: August 31, 2002

Windows System Date: August 31, 2002

1. On the Reports menu, click Practice Analysis.

2. Click the radio button for previewing the report on-screen. Click the Start button.

3. Leave the Code 1 Range boxes blank.

4. In the first Date From Range box, key *08012002*. Accept the default entry of "8/31/2002" in the second box.

5. Leave the Attending Provider Range boxes blank. Click the OK button.

6. View the report on-screen.

7. Go to the second page of the report.

8. Send the report to the printer.

9. Exit the Preview Report window.

Insurance Aging Reports

An insurance aging report permits tracking of claims filed with insurance carriers. The report lists claims that have been on file 0–30 days, 31–60 days, 61–90 days, and 91–999 days (see Figure 10-15). This information is used to follow up on overdue payments from insurance carriers. Printing the aging report and following up on overdue claims speeds the collection process. The aging begins on the date of billing. MediSoft provides three insurance aging reports: primary, secondary, and tertiary. Boxes in the Data Selection Questions dialog box for all three reports are as follows (see Figure 10-16):

Insurance Carrier 1 Range   A range of codes for insurance carriers is entered in the Insurance Carrier 1 Range boxes.

Primary Billing Date Range   A range of billing dates for the primary insurance carrier is entered in the Primary Billing Date Range boxes. The program displays the Windows System Date as the default entry in the second of these boxes.

Attending Provider Range   Codes for attending providers are entered in the Attending Provider Range boxes.

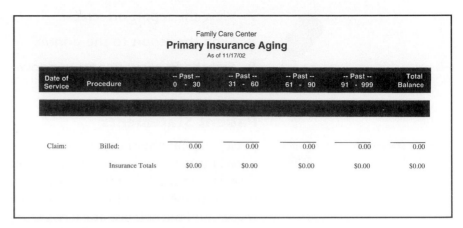

Family Care Center
Primary Insurance Aging
As of 11/17/02

Date of Service	Procedure	-- Past -- 0 - 30	-- Past -- 31 - 60	-- Past -- 61 - 90	-- Past -- 91 - 999	Total Balance
Claim:	Billed:	0.00	0.00	0.00	0.00	0.00
	Insurance Totals	$0.00	$0.00	$0.00	$0.00	$0.00

Figure 10-15 Primary Insurance Aging report.

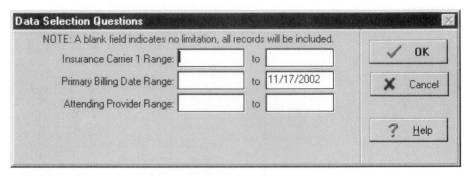

Figure 10-16 Data Selection Questions dialog box.

Exercise 10-6

Print an insurance aging report for U.S. Life for May 2003.

MediSoft Program Date: May 31, 2003

Windows System Date: May 31, 2003

1. Look up the code for U.S. Life. Click Insurance Carriers on the Lists menu. Change the entry in the Sort By box to Name. Key US in the Search box. Locate the code and write it down. Close the Insurance Carrier List dialog box.

2. On the Reports menu, click Primary Insurance Aging.

3. Click the radio button for previewing the report on-screen. Click the Start button.

4. Enter the code for U.S. Life in both of the Insurance Carrier 1 Range boxes.

5. In the first Primary Billing Date Range box, enter May 1, 2003, in MMDDCCYY format. Accept the default entry of "5/31/2003" in the second box.

6. Leave the Attending Provider Range boxes blank. Click the OK button.

7. **View the report on-screen.**

8. **Send the report to the printer.**

9. **Exit the Preview Report window.**

Patient Statements

A **patient statement** lists the amount of money a patient owes, organized by the amount of time the money has been owed, the procedures performed, and the dates the procedures were performed. The bottom of the report lists total payments, total charges, total adjustments, and the balance due (see Figure 10-17). Patient statements are printed and sent out on a regular basis to patients who have an outstanding balance.

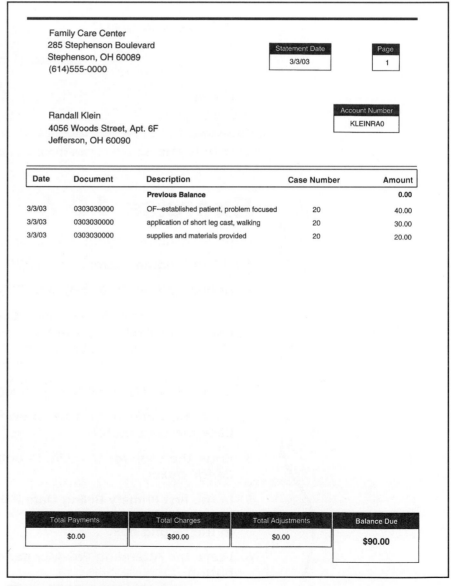

Figure 10-17 Patient statement.

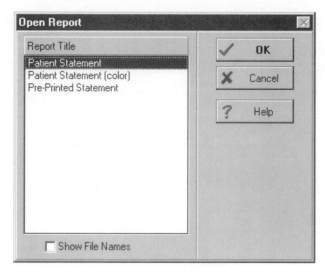

Figure 10-18 Open Report dialog box.

When Patient Statements is clicked on the Reports menu, the Open Report dialog box appears (see Figure 10-18). There are several options in the Open Report dialog box: Patient Statement, Patient Statement (Color), and Preprinted Statement. The Patient Statement option prints the standard MediSoft patient statement. The Patient Statement (Color) option prints a color version of the standard MediSoft patient statement, assuming a color printer is used. The Preprinted Statement option is chosen when a medical practice uses its own pre-printed forms to print patient statements. Like any of the standard reports in MediSoft, patient statements can be customized using MediSoft's Report Designer, discussed later in this chapter.

After the statement type is selected, the OK button is clicked. Alternatively, Patient Statement can be double-clicked. The Print Report Where? dialog box is displayed. After the choice to preview or print is made, the Data Selection Questions dialog box is displayed (see Figure 10-19). The following selections can be made:

Figure 10-19 Data Selection Questions dialog box.

Chart Number Range   In the Chart Number Range boxes, a range of chart numbers for patients is entered. If a report is needed for just one patient, that patient's chart number is entered in both boxes.

Date From Range   A range of dates is entered in the Date From Range boxes.

Billing Code Range   A range of billing codes to be included is entered in the Billing Code Range boxes.

Indicator 1 Range   If indicator codes are used by a practice, a range of codes can be entered to select only those patients who match the indicator criteria. For example, if an indicator code has been set up to track patients receiving treatment for a certain condition, it could be entered here to limit statements printed to those patients.

Patient Type Range   The Patient Type Range indicates whether the person seeing the physician is a patient or guarantor.

Attending Provider Range   Codes for attending providers are entered in the Attending Provider Range boxes.

Exercise 10-7

Print patient statements for August 2002 for those patients whose last names begin with the letters A through K.

MediSoft Program Date: August 31, 2002

Windows System Date: August 31, 2002

1. On the Reports menu, click Patient Statements.

2. In the Open Report dialog box, click Patient Statement and click the OK button.

3. Click the radio button for previewing the report on-screen. Click the Start button.

4. Key *A* in the first Chart Number Range box and *K* in the second box.

5. Enter August 1, 2002, to August 31, 2002, in the Date From Range boxes in MMDDCCYY format.

6. Leave the Billing Code Range, Indicator 1 Range, Patient Type Range, and Attending Provider Range boxes blank. Click the OK button.

7. View the report at the full width of the screen.

8. Go to the second page of the report.

9. Go to the last page of the report.

10. Send the report to the printer.

11. Exit the Preview Report window.

CUSTOM REPORTS

MediSoft has already created a number of custom reports using the built-in Report Designer. These reports include:

◆ Lists of addresses, billing codes, EMC receivers, patients, patient recalls, procedure codes, providers, and referring providers.

◆ The HCFA 1500 and the Medicare HCFA form in a variety of printer formats.

◆ Patient statements and walkout receipts.

◆ Superbills.

When Custom Report List is clicked on the Reports menu, the Open Report dialog box is displayed, listing a variety of custom reports already created in MediSoft using the Report Designer (see Figure 10-20). Additional custom reports can be created using the Report Designer. When a new custom report is created, it is added to the list of custom reports that is displayed on-screen.

The Open Report dialog box also contains six radio buttons that are used to control the list of reports displayed in the dialog box. When the All radio button is clicked, all types of custom reports are listed in the dialog box. However, when one of the other radio buttons is clicked, only reports of that style are listed. For example, if the Insurance Form radio button is clicked, only those reports that are insurance forms are listed.

To print a custom report, the title of the report is highlighted by clicking it and then the OK button is clicked. The same option that is available with standard reports for previewing the report on-screen or sending it directly to the printer is available with custom reports.

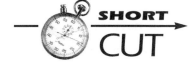
SHORT CUT

To print a custom report, double-click the report title.

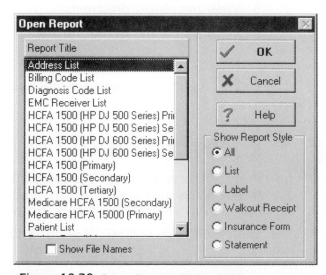

Figure 10-20 Open Report dialog box.

Exercise 10-8

Print a list of all patients.

MediSoft Program Date: August 31, 2002

Windows System Date: August 31, 2002

1. On the Reports menu, click Custom Report List.

2. Select Patient List. Click the OK button.

3. Click the radio button to preview the report on-screen. Click the Start button.

4. Leave the Chart Number Range boxes blank to select all patients.

5. Click the OK button.

6. View the report on-screen.

7. Send the report to the printer.

8. Exit the Preview Report window.

Exercise 10-9

Print a list of procedure and diagnosis codes in the database.

MediSoft Program Date: August 31, 2002

Windows System Date: August 31, 2002

1. On the Reports menu, click Custom Report List.

2. In the Show Report Style section of the dialog box, click the List radio button.

3. Select Procedure Code List. Click the OK button.

4. Click the radio button to preview the report on-screen. Click the Start button.

5. View the report on-screen.

6. Send the report to the printer.

7. Following the same steps, print a Diagnosis Code list.

8. Exit the Preview Report window.

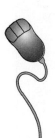

Exercise 10-10

Print a blank superbill for May 20, 2003. MediSoft uses the Windows system date for this report; the system date will be printed in the Date box on the superbill.

MediSoft Program Date: May 20, 2003

Windows System Date: May 20, 2003

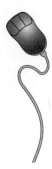

1. On the Reports menu, click Custom Report List.

2. Double-click Superbill (FCC).

3. Click the radio button to preview the report on-screen. Click the Start button.

4. View the report on-screen.

5. Send the report to the printer.

6. Exit the Preview Report window.

Using MediSoft's Report Designer allows the user maximum flexibility and control over data in the report and how they are displayed. Formatting styles include list, ledger, statement, or insurance. Reports can be created from scratch, or an existing report can be used as a starting point. The details of how to create new custom reports with the Report Designer is beyond the coverage of this text/workbook, but Exercise 10-11 offers practice working with the Report Designer to modify an existing report. The Report Designer is accessed by clicking Design Custom Reports and Bills on the Reports menu. This action causes the Report Designer window to be displayed (see Figure 10-21).

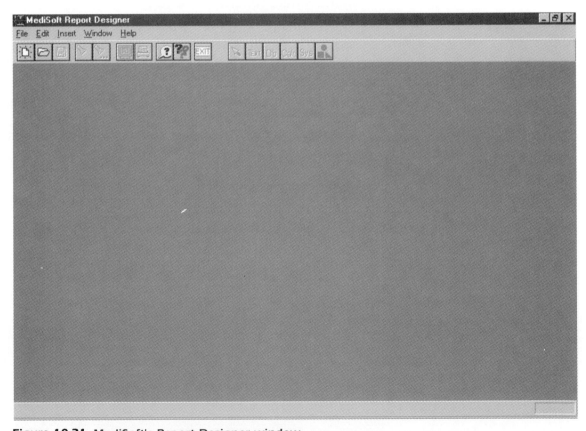

Figure 10-21 MediSoft's Report Designer window.

Exercise 10-11

Modify the Patient List report so that a work telephone number replaces a home telephone number in the report.

1. On the Reports menu, click Design Custom Reports and Bills. The Report Designer window is displayed.

2. Click Open Report on the File menu. The Open Report dialog box is displayed (see Figure 10-22).

3. Double-click Patient List in the list. The Patient List report is displayed (see Figure 10-23).

4. Notice the black band that runs across the width of the window. That band contains column labels. Double-click Phone in the black bar to edit the label to read "Work Phone." The Text Properties dialog box is displayed (see Figure 10-24).

5. Key *Work Phone* in the Text box that currently reads "Phone."

6. Since "Work Phone" contains more letters than "Phone," it is necessary to lengthen the space allotted for the label on the report so all the letters can be displayed. This is done in the section of the dialog box labeled "Size." Click in the Auto Size box to deselect that option. In the Width box, key 120 to replace the current entry (77).

7. Click the OK button. "Work Phone" is displayed on the black band where "Phone" used to be.

8. In the green band below the black band, click the Phone 11 box to select it. Then double-click the Phone 11 box to edit its contents. The Data Field Properties dialog box is displayed (see Figure 10-25 on page 214).

9. The current data box, Print Patient Phone 1, is active in the Data Field and Expressions box. Click the Edit button to change this box. The Select Data Field dialog box is displayed (see Figure 10-26 on page 214).

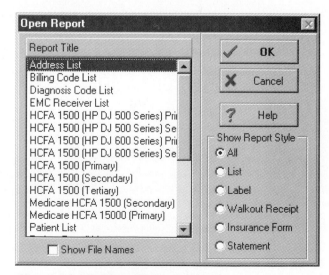

Figure 10-22 Open Report dialog box.

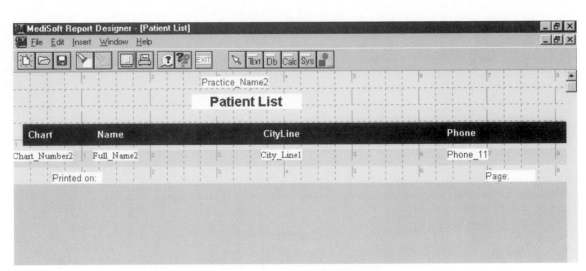

Figure 10-23 Patient List report in the MediSoft Report Designer.

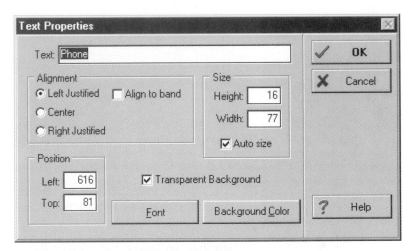

Figure 10-24 Text Properties dialog box.

10. In the Fields column, highlight Work Phone and click OK. The Data Field and Expressions box now lists Print Patient Work Phone.

11. To increase the space allotted in the report for this new value, go to the Width box and key *120*. Click the OK button. "Work Phone 1" is displayed where "Phone 11" used to be.

12. On the Report Designer File menu, click Preview Report to see how the report will look when printed. The Save Report As... dialog box is displayed.

13. Key *Patient List - Work* in the Report Title box. Click the OK button. The Data Selection Questions dialog box is displayed.

14. Leave the Chart Number Range boxes blank to select all patients for the report.

15. Click the OK button.

16. The Preview Report dialog box is displayed, showing the report.

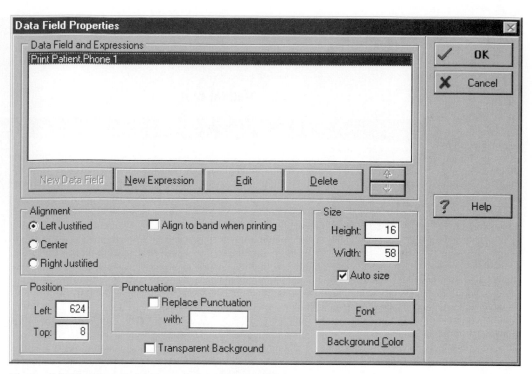

Figure 10-25 Data Field Properties dialog box.

17. Click the Print button to print the report.

18. Exit the Preview Report window.

19. Click the Close button in the top right corner of the dialog box to close the report file.

20. Click Exit on the File menu or click the Exit button on the toolbar to leave MediSoft's Report Designer.

21. Exit MediSoft.

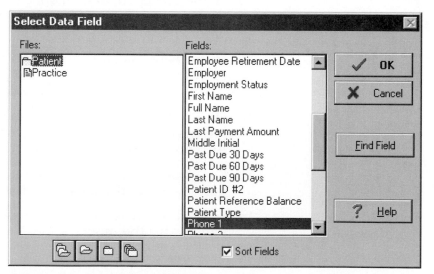

Figure 10-26 Select Data Field dialog box.

USING TERMINOLOGY

Match the terms on the left with the definitions on the right.

_____ **1.** aging report

_____ **2.** patient day sheet

_____ **3.** patient ledger

_____ **4.** patient statement

_____ **5.** procedure day sheet

a. A summary of the activity of a patient on any given day.

b. A report that lists procedures performed on a particular day and the dates, patients, document numbers, places of service, debits, and credits relating to these procedures.

c. A report that lists the amount of money owed, organized by the amount of time the money has been owed.

d. A report that lists the financial activity in each patient's account, including charges, payments, and adjustments.

e. A printed document that informs the patient of the amount of money owed.

CHECKING YOUR UNDERSTANDING

Answer the questions below in the space provided.

6. Which report can show the status of each patient's account on a separate page?

_____

_____

7. What is the name of the dialog box that has an option for including data on only those patients who fall within a certain chart number range?

_____

_____

8. Which report indicates how far past due a patient's account is?

_____

_____

CHAPTER REVIEW

9. Which entries print in a report if the boxes in the Data Selection Questions dialog box are left blank?

_____

_____

APPLYING KNOWLEDGE

Answer the questions below in the space provided.

10. One of the providers in a practice asks for a report of yesterday's transactions. How would this report be created?

_____

_____

11. A patient is unsure of whether or not she mailed a check last month for an outstanding balance on her account. How could you use MediSoft's Reports feature to help answer her question?

_____

_____

AT THE COMPUTER

Perform the following steps at the computer:

12. Print a patient ledger for John Fitzwilliams.

13. Preview an insurance aging report for Blue Cross/Blue Shield as primary carrier.

14. Print a blank superbill for September 5, 2003 for John Fitzwilliams.

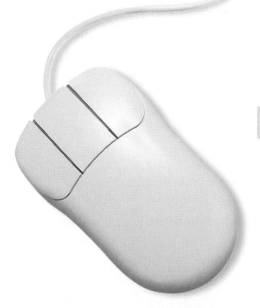

CHAPTER 11

Using Utilities

OBJECTIVES

In this chapter, you will learn how to:

◆ Make backup copies of data.

◆ View and restore backed up data.

◆ Use MediSoft's file maintenance features.

KEY TERMS

packing data   removable media device
purging data   restoring data
rebuilding files

MEDISOFT'S UTILITY FEATURES

MediSoft provides a number of built-in utilities to manage and maintain the data stored in the system. The utilities in MediSoft are used for saving/storing data, retrieving data, maintaining data files, and deleting data that is no longer needed. All MediSoft's utilities are accessed through the File menu.

Whenever information is stored on a computer, it is possible to lose data. The cause can be a machine failure, sometimes called a "hard disk crash," or the cause can be human error, such as when data is erased accidentally by pressing the wrong key. MediSoft's backup utility can minimize the amount of data that has to be reentered should a loss of data occur. If copies of computer data files, called backups (see Chapter 4), are created on a regular basis, the amount of actual data gone from a system when a data loss occurs is minimal. It is limited to the amount entered between the time of the loss and the time the last backup was performed.

Warning! Do not attempt to perform the utility functions listed in this chapter on your computer. They are for reference only. MediSoft's utility features are intended for use in a system in which data is stored on an internal hard disk. The data in this text/workbook is being stored on the Student Data Disk, a floppy disk. If the utility functions were performed, data on the Student Data Disk would be erased.

BACKING UP DATA

removable media device *a device that stores data but is not a permanent part of a computer.*

Medical offices generally have a regular schedule for backing up data. Depending on the volume of information, backups may be done as often as once a day or as infrequently as once a week. When data is backed up, it is stored on a removable media device. A **removable media device** is one that stores data but is not a permanent part of a computer. Examples of removable media devices include disks, cartridges, tapes, and CD-ROMs. Removable media devices may be stored at a location other than the office to protect them from fire or theft.

To perform a data backup in an office situation, you would complete the following steps:

1. Click Backup Data on the File menu. The MediSoft Backup dialog box is displayed (see Figure 11-1).
2. Insert the removable media device in the drive.

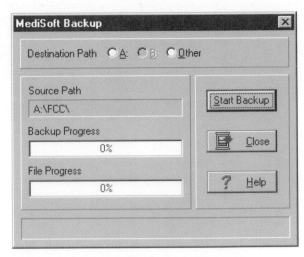

Figure 11-1 MediSoft Backup dialog box.

3. Click the Destination Path radio button that corresponds to the drive that contains the removable media device.

4. Click the Start Backup button. The backup proceeds automatically. When the backup is complete, the MediSoft Backup dialog box disappears from the screen and a "Backup complete" message is displayed. (To abort the backup process, the Close button is clicked.)

5. Eject the removable media device, and label it with the date and time of the backup and with any other information required by the medical office.

Viewing Backup Data

MediSoft provides a feature that allows a list of files on a backup device to be viewed on-screen or in a printed format. Information about the backup files is listed in the Backup View dialog box. In the top section of the dialog box, the following information is displayed: the name of the backup file and its location, the time and date it was created, the original data path, and the total number of files. The middle of the dialog box contains information about each file in the backup. File names, dates, times, original and compressed sizes, and the percentage of disk space saved by compression are listed.

To view backup data in an office situation, you would complete the following steps:

1. Click View Backup Disks on the File menu. The View Backup dialog box is displayed.

2. In the Source Path box, click the radio button for the drive that contains the disk or the device with the backup files.

3. Click the View Backup button. The Backup View dialog box is displayed (see Figure 11-2).

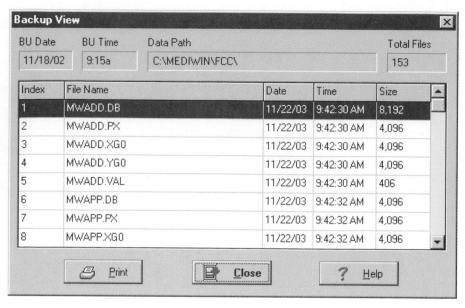

Figure 11-2 Backup View dialog box.

4. Review the information on-screen, or print it by clicking the Print button.

5. Click the Close button to exit the Backup View dialog box.

RESTORING DATA

restoring data the process of retrieving data from backup storage devices.

The process of retrieving data from backup storage devices is called **restoring data**. Data is not restored very often; only when there are serious problems with the current data is it necessary to use MediSoft's restore feature. Restoring data replaces all other data in the database. Since backup data is typically at least one day old, all the transactions, patient data, and appointments that were entered since the backup was made need to be reentered. This is one reason why it is important to print daily reports of activity in the practice. These reports can be used to reenter data when data needs to be restored.

To restore data in an office situation, you would complete the following steps:

1. Click Restore Data on the File menu. The Restore dialog box is displayed (see Figure 11-3).

2. Insert the removable media device that contains the backup data in the drive.

3. Click the Source Path radio button that corresponds to the drive that contains the removable media device.

4. Click the Start Restore button. (To abort the Restore process, click the Close button.)

5. The restore proceeds automatically. When the process is complete, the Restore dialog box disappears from the screen.

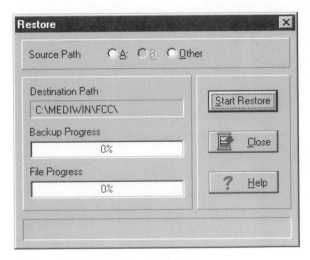

Figure 11-3 Restore dialog box.

FILE MAINTENANCE UTILITIES

MediSoft provides four features to assist in maintaining data files stored in a system. These four features are found on tabs in the File Maintenance dialog box (see Figure 11-4):

◆ Rebuild Files

◆ Pack Data

◆ Recalculate Balances

◆ Purge Data

The dialog box is accessed by clicking File Maintenance on the File menu.

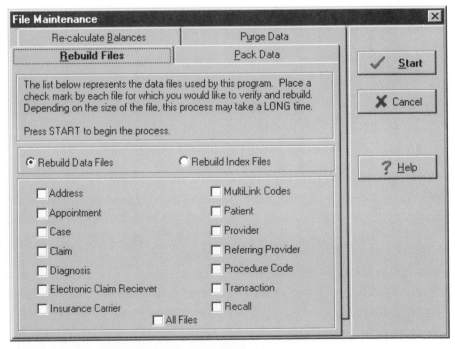

Figure 11-4 File Maintenance dialog box.

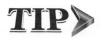 **TIP**

If the medical office's database is large, MediSoft's utilities may take a long time to finish. For this reason, it is usually a good idea to use the utility functions at the end of the day or when the system will not be needed for a while.

Rebuilding Files

rebuilding files *a process that checks and verifies data and corrects any internal problems with the data.*

Rebuilding files is a process that checks and verifies data and corrects any internal problems with the data. The rebuild does not check or verify the content of the data. For example, the system will not check whether John Fitzwilliams paid $50 on his last visit. Rebuilding does not change the content of any data files. To keep files working efficiently, files should be rebuilt about once a month. Files to be rebuilt are selected from the list of files in the Rebuild Files tab (see Figure 11-5). If the database is large, rebuilding files could take a long time.

There are two radio buttons on the Rebuild Files tab: Rebuild Data Files and Rebuild Index Files. In most cases, it is appropriate to accept the default of Rebuild Data Files.

To rebuild files in Medisoft in an office, you would complete the following steps:

1. Click File Maintenance on the File menu. The File Maintenance dialog box is displayed with the Rebuild Files tab active.
2. Click in each check mark box next to the files that are to be verified and rebuilt.

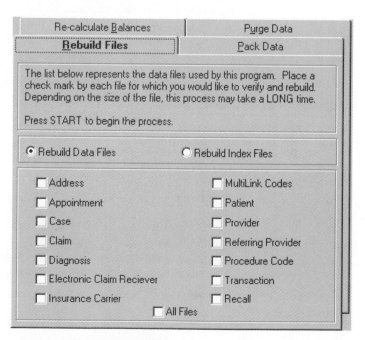

Figure 11-5 Rebuild Files tab.

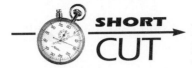

If all files are to be rebuilt, click the All Files box at the bottom of the list of files. This saves the time it would take to click a box for every MediSoft file.

3. Click the Start button. The Confirm dialog box is displayed with the message "All of the checked file processes will be performed. Do you want to continue?" Click the OK button to continue. (Clicking the Cancel button aborts the process.)

4. The rebuild process is performed automatically. When the process is complete, the message, "All checked file processes are complete," is displayed.

Packing Data

When data is deleted in MediSoft, the system empties the data from the record but keeps the empty slot in the database so it is available when new data needs to be entered in the system. For example, if a patient were deleted in the Patient List dialog box, the system would delete all the records pertaining to that patient but would maintain an empty slot in the patient database. Then, the next time a new patient is entered, the data for the new patient would occupy the vacant slot in the database. In cases in which there is not much space available on the hard disk, it is sometimes desirable to delete the vacant slots to make more disk space available. The deletion of vacant slots from the database is known as **packing data**. Data for packing can be selected from the list of files in the Pack Data tab (see Figure 11-6). (Only transaction files with a zero balance can be deleted.) If the database is large, packing data can take a long time.

packing data the deletion of vacant slots from a database.

Re-calculate Balances	Purge Data
Rebuild Files	**Pack Data**

The list below represents the data files used by this program. Place a check mark by each file for which you would like to remove deleted data. Depending on the size of the file, this process may take a LONG time.

Press OK to start the process.

- [ ] Address
- [ ] Appointment
- [ ] Case
- [ ] Claim
- [ ] Diagnosis
- [ ] Electronic Claim Reciever
- [ ] Insurance Carrier
- [ ] MultiLink Codes
- [ ] Patient
- [ ] Provider
- [ ] Referring Provider
- [ ] Procedure Code
- [ ] Transaction
- [ ] Recall
- [ ] All Files

Figure 11-6 Pack Data tab.

To pack files in an office situation, you would complete the following steps:

1. Click File Maintenance on the File menu. The File Maintenance dialog box is displayed with the Rebuild Files tab active. Make the Pack Data tab active.

2. Click in each check mark box next to the files that are to have deleted data removed.

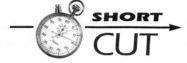

If all files are to be checked for deleted data, click the All Files box at the bottom of the list of files.

3. Click the Start button. The Confirm dialog box is displayed with the message, "All of the checked file processes will be performed. Do you want to continue?" Click the OK button to continue. (Clicking the Cancel button aborts the process.)

4. The pack process is performed automatically. When the process is complete, the message, "All checked file processes are complete," is displayed.

Recalculating Patient Balances

As transaction entries are changed or deleted, there are times when the balance listed on-screen is not accurate. To update balances to reflect the most recent changes made to the data, the Re-calculate Balances feature is used. This feature is accessed through the Re-calculate Balances tab on the File Maintenance dialog box (see Figure 11-7).

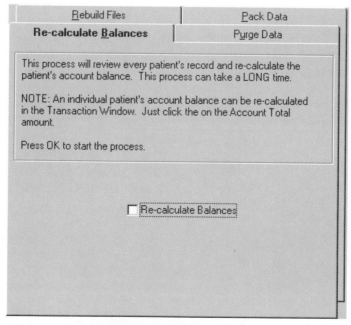

Figure 11-7 Re-calculate Balances tab.

When balances are recalculated, the system reviews every patient's data and recalculates the balances. The process of recalculating balances can be time-consuming. Individual patient balances can be recalculated in the Transaction Entry dialog box by clicking the Account Total column.

To recalculate balances in an office situation, you would complete the following steps:

1. Click File Maintenance on the File menu. The File Maintenance dialog box is displayed with the Rebuild Files tab active. Make the Recalculate Balances tab active.

2. Click to place a check mark in the Recalculate Balances box.

3. Click the Start button. The Confirm dialog box is displayed with the message, "All of the checked file processes will be performed. Do you want to continue?" Click the OK button to continue. (Clicking the Cancel button aborts the process.)

4. The recalculate process is performed automatically. When the process is complete, the message, "All checked file processes are complete," is displayed.

Purging Data

purging data the process of deleting files of patients who are no longer seen by a provider in a practice.

The process of deleting files of patients who are no longer seen by a provider in a practice is called **purging data**. Purging data frees space on the computer and permits the system to run more efficiently. *However, purging should be done with great caution.* Once data is purged from the system, it cannot be retrieved, except from a backup file. As a safety precaution, always perform a backup before purging.

The Purge Data tab offers several options (see Figure 11-8 on page 226). Data can be purged for appointments, claims, or for closed cases. Appointment and claim data are purged by date. A cutoff date is entered. MediSoft deletes all data up to that date. For example, if all the data entered prior to December 31, 1995, is to be purged, that date would be entered as the cutoff date. Data entered in cases that have been closed is purged by clicking the check box labeled "Purge Closed Cases."

To purge data in an office situation, you would complete the following steps:

1. Click File Maintenance on the File menu. The File Maintenance dialog box is displayed with the Rebuild Files tab active. Make the Purge Data tab active.

2. Click in each check mark box next to the files that are to be purged. If Appointments or Claims are being purged, enter a cutoff date in the Cutoff Dates box. Dates are entered in the usual MMDDYY format.

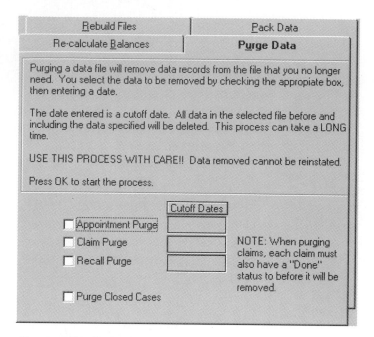

Rebuild Files	Pack Data
Re-calculate Balances	**Purge Data**

Purging a data file will remove data records from the file that you no longer need. You select the data to be removed by checking the appropiate box, then entering a date.

The date entered is a cutoff date. All data in the selected file before and including the data specified will be deleted. This process can take a LONG time.

USE THIS PROCESS WITH CARE!! Data removed cannot be reinstated.

Press OK to start the process.

Cutoff Dates

☐ Appointment Purge

☐ Claim Purge

☐ Recall Purge

NOTE: When purging claims, each claim must also have a "Done" status to before it will be removed.

☐ Purge Closed Cases

Figure 11-8 Purge Data tab.

3. Click the Start button. The Confirm dialog box is displayed with the message, "All of the checked file processes will be performed. Do you want to continue?" Click the OK button to continue. (Clicking the Cancel button aborts the process.)

4. The purge process is performed automatically. When the process is complete, the message "All checked file processes are complete," is displayed.

CHAPTER REVIEW

USING TERMINOLOGY

Match the terms on the left with the definitions on the right.

_____ **1.** packing data

_____ **2.** purging data

_____ **3.** rebuilding files

_____ **4.** removable media device

_____ **5.** restoring data

a. A device that stores data but is not a permanent part of a computer.

b. A process that checks and verifies data and corrects any internal problems with the data.

c. The process of retrieving data from backup storage devices.

d. The deletion of vacant data slots from a database.

e. The process of deleting files of patients who are no longer seen by a provider of a practice.

CHECKING YOUR UNDERSTANDING

Answer the questions below in the space provided.

6. Why is it important to back up data regularly?

_____

_____

7. Why is extra caution required when purging data?

_____

_____

8. When is a data restore performed?

_____

_____

9. In MediSoft, where are the two places a patient's balance can be recalculated?

_____

_____

APPLYING KNOWLEDGE

Answer the question below in the space provided.

10. You come in to work on a Monday morning and find the office computer is not working. The system manager informs everyone that the computer's hard disk crashed, and that all data that was not backed up is lost. What do you do?

_____

_____

_____

_____

Simulations

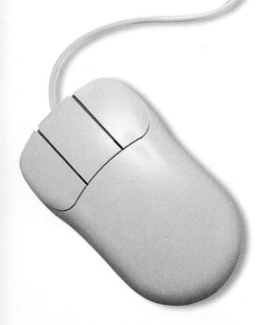

CHAPTER 12

Handling Patient Records and Transactions

WHAT YOU NEED TO KNOW

To complete the simulations in this chapter, you need to know how to:

◆ Locate patient information.
◆ Change the Windows System Date and the MediSoft Program Date.
◆ Assign a new chart number and enter information on a new patient.
◆ Add a new case record for a patient.
◆ Change information on an established patient.
◆ Add an insurance company to the database.
◆ Enter procedures, charges, and diagnoses.
◆ Record payments from patients.
◆ Print walkout receipts.

All office personnel at the Family Care Center (FCC) know how to input patient information in the Patient/Guarantor dialog box and in the Case dialog box. Whenever possible, all information for both dialog boxes is entered into the computer as soon as patients complete the handwritten information sheet and hand it to the receptionist. On busy days, however, or when the office is understaffed because one of the medical assistants is sick or on vacation, input operations may be delayed.

SIMULATION 12-1: INPUTTING PATIENT INFORMATION

For this simulation, you need Source Documents 8–12.

It is Monday, November 17, 2003. You are a records/billing clerk at the Family Care Center. On your desk is a small pile of information sheets and superbills from Friday afternoon, November 14. You decide to input all patient information first and then go back and record the transactions. First, you arrange the papers alphabetically:

Battistuta

Brooks

Hsu

Syzmanski

Then you begin.

On the File menu, click Set Program Date. A pop-up calendar is displayed in the lower right corner of the screen. Select November 14, 2003, as the date, using the drop-down lists for month and year. Click the check mark when you have selected the date. November 14, 2003, is displayed on the status bar.

Patient 1: Anthony Battistuta

Record the address and phone number changes that are written on Mr. Battistuta's superbill (Source Document 8).

1. Click Patients/Guarantors and Cases on the Lists menu. The Patient List dialog box is displayed.

2. Select Anthony Battistuta from the list of patients.

3. Click the Edit Patient button. The Patient/Guarantor dialog box is displayed, with the Name, Address tab active.

4. Enter the new address and phone number.

5. Click the Save button.

Patient 2: Lawana Brooks

You can see from the superbill (Source Document 9) that Ms. Brooks is an established patient. There are no changes to be made for her in the Patient/Guarantor dialog box. The work you need to do must take place in the Case dialog box. Ms. Brooks has had an accident at work, so a new case Workers' Compensation must be created.

1. After saving the changes for Mr. Battistuta in the Patient/ Guarantor dialog box, the Patient List dialog box is redisplayed.

2. In the list of patients, click the listing for Brooks to select her as the patient. From the list of cases, click the one for ankle sprain. (You will not enter new information in the ankle sprain case; instead, you will copy information from the ankle sprain case to create a new case.)

3. Click the Copy Case button to copy the information from the existing case into a new case. A duplicate case is displayed.

4. Edit the information in the case to reflect the information relevant to the new case by changing the following boxes:

Personal Tab
Description: Workers' Compensation

Diagnosis Tab
Diagnosis 1: 841.0 sprain or strain of radical collateral
Diagnosis 2: E885 fall on same level from slipping
Diagnosis 3: E849.3 industrial place and premises
(These codes must be added to the Diagnosis Codes database.)

Condition Tab
Injury/Illness/LMP Date: 11/14/03 (Enter Friday's date in MMDDYY format.)
Employment Related: ✓
Emergency: ✓
Accident Related to: Yes
State: OH
Nature of: Work Injury/Non-collision
Workers' Compensation Return to Work Indicator: Limited
Workers' Compensation Percent of Disability: 20

5. Save your work.

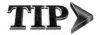 When entering information on different tabs within a dialog box, it is not necessary to click the Save button after completing each tab. However, the Save button must be clicked once all the tabs are complete, before exiting the dialog box.

Patient 3: Edwin Hsu

1. The information you need to make the necessary changes to the Patient/Guarantor dialog box for Edwin Hsu is on Source Document 10. The new insurance company, Midwest Select, is not on the patient information form nor is it in FCC's database. Edwin Hsu does not have his insurance card. You look up Midwest Select in the phone book, find the correct ZIP Code on

the map in the front of the phone book, and call the insurance company to find out what percentage of charges are covered by the plan. Midwest pays 80 percent after a $500 deductible.

2. After saving the new case for Brooks, you are in the Patient List dialog box. Select Edwin Hsu, and click the Edit Patient button.

3. Move to the Street box, and enter the new address.

4. Move to the Phones 1 box and enter the new phone number.

5. Save the information you just entered.

6. Now the new insurance carrier must be added to the database. From the Lists menu, click Insurance Carriers.

7. The Insurance Carrier List dialog box is displayed.

8. There are 15 insurance companies in FCC's database. Midwest Select will be No. 16. Click the New button to add information for Midwest.

9. Enter the information below in the correct boxes:

Address Tab
Code: 16
Name: Midwest Select
Street: 1245 Mohawk Lane
City: Columbus
State: OH
ZIP Code: 60625
Phone: (614) 555-1211
Practice ID: 12345678

Options Tab
Plan Name: Midwest Select
Type: Other
Procedure Code Set: 1
Diagnosis Code Set: 1
Signature on File: Signature on file
Default Billing Method: Electronic
Print PINs on Forms: Leave blank

EMC, Codes Tab
EMC Receiver: 0000—National Data Corporation
EMC Payor Number: 50678
EMC Sub ID: 5034
NDC Record Code: 01

10. Click the Save button. Midwest Select is now displayed on the list of insurance carriers.

11. Close the Insurance Carrier List dialog box. The Patient List dialog box is still displayed. Edwin Hsu is still the selected patient.

12. Create a new case for Edwin Hsu by copying his existing case.

13. Edit the information in the copied case to reflect the information relevant to the new case by changing the following boxes:

Personal Tab
Description: Acute sinusitis

Diagnosis Tab
Diagnosis 1: 461.9

Policy 1 Tab
Insurance 1: 16 - Midwest Select
Accept Assignment Transaction Default: ✓
Policy Number: 51249
Group Number: 256
Copayment Amount: 0
Insurance Coverage Percents by Service Classification: 80

Condition Tab
Injury/Illness/LMP Date: 11/14/03
Illness Indicator: Illness

14. Save the file.

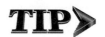 Do not change the insurance carrier in the urinary tract infection case for Edwin Hsu, because at the time he was treated for that condition, Hsu was covered by East Ohio PPO, not Midwest Select.

Patient 4: Hannah Syzmanski

Use Source Documents 11 and 12 to enter information on a new patient, Hannah Syzmanski. Hannah is the daughter of Michael and Debra Syzmanski, who are patients of Dr. Dana Banu. Hannah has been seeing her own doctor, a pediatrician, but is now switching to the Family Care Center.

1. Go to the Patient List dialog box, and click the New Patient button.

2. Key *SYZMAHA0* in the Chart Number box.

3. Complete the boxes for name, address, phone, birth date, sex, and Social Security number.

4. In the Other Information tab, complete the boxes as follows:

Type: Patient

Assigned Provider: 6 - Dana Banu

Patient ID #2: Leave blank

Signature on File: ✓

Signature Date: November 14, 2003

5. Save your work.

6. Click the Case radio button to make the Case portion of the Patient List dialog box active.

7. Click the New Case button to open a new Case dialog box.

8. Complete the tabs in the Case dialog box as follows:

Personal Tab

Description: Complete physical

Guarantor: SYZMADEØ Syzmanski, Debra

Student Status: Full time

Account Tab

Referring Provider: 13 - Harold Gearhart, MD

Diagnosis Tab

Diagnosis 1: V70.0

Allergies and Notes: Bee stings

Policy 1 Tab

When you attempt to complete the Policy 1 tab, you notice that Hannah has not filled in her insurance company, but since she is covered by her mother's insurance, you know that information will be easy to find. First save your work on Hannah's case. Then open the Case dialog box for the urinary tract infection case for Debra Syzmanski, and go to the Policy 1 tab. Use the information on that tab to fill in the missing insurance data for Hannah Syzmanski. (The information is U.S. Life, accept assignment, 80 percent coverage, Policy Number 45539G, Group Number 0679.)

When completing the Policy 1 tab for Hannah, remember to list Debra Syzmanski in the Insured 1 box and to click Child in the Relationship to Insured box.

9. Save your work.

SIMULATION 12-2: AN EMERGENCY VISIT

You will need Source Document 13 for this simulation.

It is still Monday morning, November 17. Carlos Lopez has just seen Dr. McGrath on an emergency basis. Mr. Lopez thought he was having a heart attack. Fortunately, Dr. McGrath has determined that he was just suffering from heart palpitations. Mr. Lopez has handed you the superbill for his visit and wants to pay his part of the charge in cash. (For the purposes of this simulation, assume that FCC uses MediSoft to generate patient receipts.) You need to enter the appropriate information from the superbill in the Transaction Entry dialog box, tell Mr. Lopez how much he owes, accept his payment, and print a walkout receipt. Make sure all transaction information is properly recorded in the database.

1. Change the Windows System Date and the MediSoft Program Date to November 17, 2003.

2. From the Patient List dialog box, create a new case for Carlos Lopez by copying the information in the case that already exists.

3. Enter the following information:

   Personal Tab
   Description: Heart palpitations

   Diagnosis Tab
   Diagnosis 1: V65.5

   Condition Tab
   Injury/Illness/LMP Date: 11/17/03
   Illness Indicator: Illness
   First Consultation Date: 11/17/03
   Emergency: ✓

4. Save your work.

5. Click Enter Transactions on the Activities menu.

6. Select Mr. Lopez in the Chart box.

7. Select heart palpitations in the Case box.

8. Click the New button to create a new transaction. The Charge tab is active.

9. Verify that 11/17/03 is displayed in the Dates boxes.

10. In the Document box, you have the option of accepting the default document number, which is a variation of the day's date,

or using a number of your own choosing. FCC uses the default document numbering system, so accept the displayed number.

11. Enter the first procedure number checked on the superbill: 93000. Press the Tab key. "60.00" is automatically entered in the Amount box.

12. Accept the default entries in the POS and Units boxes.

13. Save the transaction and open a new transaction by clicking the Save/Open button.

14. Enter the other procedure number from the superbill: 99212. Press the Tab key. Verify that 40.00 is displayed in the Amount box.

15. Click the Save/Close button to save the transaction and return to the main Transaction Entry dialog box.

16. Look at the left side of the dialog box, where the amount the insurance carrier is responsible for is listed and the amount Mr. Lopez owes is listed. You tell Mr. Lopez that his part of the payment is $20.00. He gives you cash.

17. To record Mr. Lopez's payment, click the New button and go to the Payment tab.

18. If the date (11/17/03) and document number (0311170000) are correct, accept them.

19. In the Pay Code box, select the option that reads "01 - patient payment, cash."

20. In the Who Paid box, select Carlos Lopez.

21. Key *Cash Payment* in the Description box.

22. Key *20* in the Amount box and press the Tab key.

23. To apply the payment to charges, click the Apply Payment to Charges button.

24. Click the This Payment box, key 20, and press the Tab key.

25. Click the Close button.

26. Click the Save/Close button to return to the initial Transaction Entry dialog box. Notice that the payment is now listed under the charge at the bottom of the list of transactions, and that the amount owed by Mr. Lopez is now listed as 0.00.

27. Click the Print Receipt button to print a walkout receipt.

SIMULATION 12-3: INPUTTING TRANSACTION DATA

For this simulation, you need Source Documents 8, 9, 10, and 12.

You are now ready to record the transactions from Friday's four superbills. Before you begin, set the MediSoft Program Date and the Windows System Date to November 14, 2003.

Anthony Battistuta

1. Click Enter Transactions on the Activities menu.

2. Select Anthony Battistuta in the Chart box.

3. Verify that Diabetes is displayed to the right of the Case box.

4. Record the procedures, one at a time.

5. Save your work.

Lawana Brooks

Follow essentially the same procedures as you did for Anthony Battistuta. You need to record the date and procedures and save your work. Close the Transaction Entry dialog box.

Edwin Hsu

Follow essentially the same procedures as you did for Anthony Battistuta. You need to record the date and procedure, and then Mr. Hsu's payment. Apply the payment to the charges, and save your work.

Hannah Syzmanski

Follow essentially the same procedures as you did for Anthony Battistuta. You need to record the date and procedure and save your work.

Change in Lawana Brooks's Transaction File

You discover a note that had been attached to Lawana Brooks's superbill, saying, "Charge for visit should be $50—professional courtesy." Make the change in Ms. Brooks's file.

1. Go to the Transaction Entry dialog box. Select the line that contains the procedure charge with an error, and click the Edit button.

2. In the Amount box, change 100.00 to 50.00. Press the Tab key.

3. Save your work.

SIMULATION 12-4: CHRISTOPHER PALMER

For this simulation, you need Source Documents 14 and 15.

The date is November 17, 2003. Change the MediSoft and Windows dates to November 17, 2003. Enter patient information and all transactions for Christopher Palmer, a new patient of Dr. Beach.

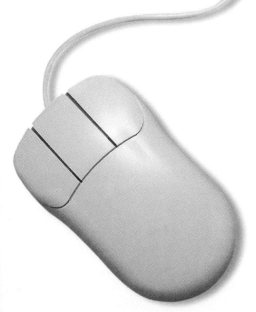

13 Setting Up Appointments

WHAT YOU NEED TO KNOW

To complete the simulations in this chapter, you need to know how to:

◆ Start Office Hours.

◆ Move around in the schedule.

◆ Enter appointments.

◆ Change appointment information.

◆ Move or copy an appointment.

◆ Schedule a recall appointment.

◆ Create a new case record for a patient.

◆ Change a transaction record.

The Family Care Center uses Office Hours as the primary tool for recording appointments. For the simulations in this chapter, assume that you are the front-desk receptionist/clerk and are responsible for most of the Center's scheduling tasks. Remember, you can access Office Hours at any time, no matter what you are working on. For example, suppose you are typing a letter for one of the doctors and you get a phone call from a patient who wants to make an appointment. All you have to do is click the Start button on the task bar; select Programs—MediSoft, and then Office Hours; enter the appointment; exit Office Hours; and return to your word processing program. Office Hours can also be accessed from within MediSoft, either by clicking the shortcut button or by clicking Appointment Book on the Activities menu.

SIMULATION 13-1: MAKING AN APPOINTMENT CHANGE

It is still Monday, November 17, 2003. Carlos Lopez has just called to say that he has lost his appointment card and cannot remember what time his appointment is on December 1. He thinks there may be a scheduling conflict with a meeting he has that day. If the appointment is in the morning, he wants you to change it to 2:00 p.m. that same day. If the 2:00 p.m. slot is not available, he needs to make the appointment for the next day at the earliest possible time.

1. Access Office Hours. The current date (11/17/03) is displayed in the calendar and on the schedule.

2. Go to December 2003.

3. Move to December 1 on the calendar. (Since Mr. Lopez's doctor is Patricia McGrath, and Katherine Yan is the provider listed in the Provider box, you need to change the provider before continuing.)

4. Locate Mr. Lopez's appointment.

5. Check to see whether 2:00 p.m., the time he wanted to change the appointment to, is available.

6. Since 2:00 is not available, move to December 2 on the calendar. Dr. McGrath has no appointments scheduled on December 2.

7. Go back to December 1. Move Mr. Lopez's appointment from December 1 to December 2 at 9:00 a.m. (If you do not remember how to move an appointment, see Chapter 8.)

SIMULATION 13-2: JUGGLING SCHEDULES

Mrs. Jackson's sister is on the phone. She will be taking care of the Jackson twins on Saturday, December 13, 2003, and she needs to make an appointment for both of them for a physical and a tetanus shot sometime after 9:00 a.m. That is the only day they can come in, so she hopes you can accommodate her. She does not remember the name of their doctor.

1. Find out who the twins' doctor is by calling up the Patient/Guarantor dialog box for either of the twins. Select the Other Information tab, and check the Assigned Provider box.

2. Go into Office Hours, and check Dr. Dana Banu's schedule for December 13. She is booked solid from 9:00 a.m. until she leaves at 1:00 p.m.

3. Check two other physicians—Dr. McGrath and Dr. Beach. Dr. McGrath will not be in the office on December 13. However, Dr. Robert Beach has several open slots. Book Darnell in the 10:30 time slot and Tyrone in the 10:45 a.m. slot.

SIMULATION 13-3: ADDING PATIENTS TO THE RECALL LIST

Darnell and Tyrone Jackson need to be called back for follow-up appointments in six months. Add both of them to the Recall list for six months from December 13, 2003.

1. Click Patient Recall on the Lists menu. The Patient Recall List dialog box is displayed.

2. Click the New button.

3. Enter June 14, 2003 in the Recall Date box, using the MMDDYY format.

4. Select Dr. Dana Banu in the Provider box.

5. Key the first six letters of Darnell Jackson's chart number in the Chart box. Press the Tab key.

6. In the Message box, key *Six month follow-up appointment needed.*

7. Verify that the Call radio button in the Recall Status box is selected.

8. Click the Save button to save the entry.

9. Repeat the steps to add Tyrone Jackson to the Patient Recall List.

10. Close the Patient Recall List dialog box.

SIMULATION 13-4: DIANE HSU AND MICHAEL SYZMANSKI

For this simulation, you will need Source Documents 16 and 17.

It is still Monday, November 17. Diane Hsu and Michael Syzmanski are leaving the office after their appointments. Use the information on Source Documents 16 and 17 to perform the following tasks:

1. Create new cases for both patients by copying existing cases.

   For Mrs. Hsu, complete the Personal, Diagnosis, and Policy 1 tabs. When completing the Policy 1 tab for Mrs. Hsu, remember that Mrs. Hsu's husband changed insurance carriers to Midwest Select, and since Mrs. Hsu is covered under her husband's policy, the new insurance company information must be used:

   Insured 1: HSUEDWI∅ - Hsu, Edwin
   Relationship to Insured: Spouse
   Insurance 1: Midwest Select
   Accept Assignment Transaction Default: ✓
   Policy Number: 51249
   Group Number: 256
   Copayment Amount: 0
   Insurance Coverage Percents by Service Classification: 80

   For Mr. Syzmanski, complete the Personal and Diagnosis tabs.

2. Record the charges and payments in the Transaction Entry dialog box. For Mrs. Hsu, you need to enter the $15 charge for procedure 90782. The system does not automatically enter the charge, since charges for injections vary at FCC.

   Mrs. Hsu pays $15 in cash; this payment should be applied to the charge for procedure 87072.

   Michael Syzmanski pays $34 with Check 319; this payment should be applied to the charge for procedure 45378. Record the payments and apply the payments to the charges.

3. Print walkout receipts.

4. Make the appointment indicated on Mrs. Hsu's superbill, using Office Hours. Do not exit MediSoft.

SIMULATION 13-5: CHANGING A TRANSACTION RECORD

Just as you finish making Mrs. Hsu's appointment, Dr. Robert Beach comes to the desk to say that he thinks he forgot to put down on the superbill the injection of penicillin he gave Christopher Palmer. He asks you to check and add the charge ($15) if necessary.

1. Go to the Transaction Entry dialog box. Check through the entries to find out whether the charge was entered. (It was not.)

2. Enter the new charge.

3. Save your work.

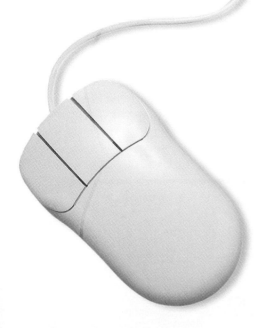

CHAPTER

14 Printing Superbills, Lists, and Reports

WHAT YOU NEED TO KNOW

To complete the simulations in this chapter, you need to know how to:

◆ Create a patient ledger.
◆ Create a day sheet report.
◆ Create a patient aging report.
◆ Create an insurance aging report.
◆ Understand what aging means, in an accounting sense.
◆ Enter transactions.
◆ Print a superbill.
◆ Print an appointment list.
◆ Print a patient ledger report.

Because MediSoft is an accounting package, its most powerful features involve computerized manipulation of account data for patients. MediSoft uses information in the system to produce reports on any facet of patients' or insurers' accounts and to generate bills for patients and insurance companies. For example, as long as the office personnel in the Family Care Center have entered transactions correctly and have performed basic accounting procedures, the MediSoft program can be used to print current reports on the center's finances. You can print a report showing details of a day's transactions for any one of the center's physicians or for all physicians. You can print a report of late accounts for a particular patient, for all patients, for one insurance company, or for all insurance companies.

Before starting the simulations in this chapter, you should understand some basic aspects of medical office accounting procedures.

Every medical office must keep a daily record of charges and payments made for every patient of every doctor. For charges, the record usually includes the name of the patient, the type of service provided, and the amount of the charge. For payments, the record usually includes the name of the patient whose account is being credited and the amount of the payment. Whereas day sheets record information on charges and payments for a single day, ledgers show all current information up to and including the date shown on the ledger.

As the name suggests, aging reports show clearly how long unpaid charges have been due. In MediSoft, aging reports are divided into four columns, showing, in order, accounts that are currently due, accounts that have been due for 31–60 days, accounts that have been due for 61–90 days, and accounts that have been due for more than 90 days.

SIMULATION 14-1: FINDING A PATIENT'S BALANCE

It is still Monday, November 17. Debra Syzmanski calls. She is planning to come in to pay her daughter Hannah's charges for Friday's visit. Rather than bring her checkbook, she wants to write a check before she leaves home. How can you find the amount she owes?

MediSoft Program Date: November 17, 2003
Windows System Date: November 17, 2003

1. On the Activities menu, click Enter Transactions.

2. In the Chart box, select Hannah Syzmanski's chart number.

3. Verify that the "Complete physical" case is active in the Case box, and that the transaction listed at the bottom of the dialog box is for Friday, November 14.

4. Look at the left side of the dialog box, where the information about financial responsibility is listed. Notice that the insurance carrier, U.S. Life, is responsible for $160 (80 percent of the total bill) and Debra Syzmanski, as guarantor, is responsible for $40 (20 percent of the total bill).

SIMULATION 14-2: PRINTING A SCHEDULE

Print the appointment schedule for Dr. Dana Banu for Saturday, December 13, 2003.

MediSoft Program Date: December 13, 2003
Windows System Date: December 13, 2003

1. Open Office Hours.

2. Select Dr. Dana Banu as the Provider.

3. Go to December 13, 2003 in the calendar.

4. Click Print Appointment List on the File menu.

SIMULATION 14-3: PRINTING SUPERBILLS

Print three superbills.

MediSoft Program Date: November 17, 2003
Windows System Date: November 17, 2003

1. On the Reports menu, click Custom Report List.

2. In the Open Report dialog box, select Superbill (FCC).

3. Click the OK button.

4. In the Print Report Where? dialog box, choose the option that sends the report directly to the printer.

5. Click the Start button.

6. In the Print dialog box, key 3 in the Copies box to print three copies of the report.

7. Click the OK button.

SIMULATION 14-4: PRINTING DAY SHEET REPORTS

Before MediSoft can generate a day sheet, the day's transactions must be recorded in the MediSoft database.

MediSoft Program Date: November 17, 2003
Windows System Date: November 17, 2003

1. Use the three superbills you printed in Simulation 14-3 as source documents for the charges and payments for Sheila Giles, Raji Patel, and Nancy Stern. All patients have appointments on November 17, 2003. Before entering any data into MediSoft, write these procedures on the superbills:

   Giles, office visit, established patient, expanded
   Patel, office visit, established patient, problem focused
   Stern, office visit, established patient, problem focused

Write in these codes for diagnoses:

Giles, 760.0
Patel, 760.0
Stern, 466.0

2. Using the procedures and codes for diagnoses you just wrote in on the superbills, enter the transactions.

3. Enter the following payments:

Giles, $16, Check 1121
Patel, $4 cash
Stern, $8 cash

4. Be sure to save your work.

Patient day sheets and procedure day sheets can be viewed and/or printed using options on the Reports menu.

Creating a Patient Day Sheet Report

1. On the Reports menu, click Patient Day Sheet.

2. Select the option to preview the report on-screen. Click the Start button.

3. Leave the Chart Number Range boxes blank, to include all patients.

4. Accept the default of 11/17/2003 in the Date Created Range boxes.

5. Leave both Date From Range boxes and the Attending Provider Range boxes blank.

6. Click the OK button.

7. The patient day sheet report is displayed on-screen.

8. Close the Preview Report window.

Creating a Procedure Day Sheet Report

1. On the Reports menu, click Procedure Day Sheet.

2. Select the option to preview the report on-screen. Click the Start button.

3. Leave the Code 1 Range boxes blank.

4. Use the Tab key to move to the first Date Created Range box. Delete the default date.

5. Use the Tab key to move to the second Date Created Range box. Delete the default date.

6. Key *11172003* in both of the Date From Range boxes.

7. Leave the Attending Provider boxes blank.

8. Click the OK button.

9. The procedure day sheet report appears on-screen.

10. Close the Preview Report window.

SIMULATION 14-5: CREATING A PATIENT AGING REPORT

Print a patient aging report as a first step in the billing process. The aging report shows which accounts are overdue and how long they have been overdue.

MediSoft Program Date: December 31, 2003
Windows System Date: December 31, 2003

1. On the Report menu, click Patient Aging.

2. Select the option to preview the report on the screen. Click the Start button.

3. Leave all data selection fields blank except the second Date From Range box, which displays the default date of 12/31/2003.

4. View the report.

5. Close the Preview Report window.

SIMULATION 14-6: RECORDING A PAYMENT FOR A PAST TRANSACTION

Lawana Brooks has come in with her check for $22.60 (Check 316). Record this payment. Use November 24, 2003 as the MediSoft Program Date and the Windows System Date.

SIMULATION 14-7: STEWART ROBERTSON

You need Source Document 18 for this simulation, which consists of three parts. For the first part, assume that it is still November 17, 2003. A new patient of Dr. Beach, Stewart Robertson, has stopped by to fill out a patient information form, but he wants an appointment for December, specifically for the second Saturday of the month, if possible. He needs an appointment and an ECG (30 minutes).

Part One - November 17, 2003

MediSoft Program Date: November 17, 2003
Windows System Date: November 17, 2003

1. Using Source Document 18, enter the patient information for Mr. Robertson, a new patient of Dr. Robert Beach. Complete the Patient/Guarantor dialog box and the Case dialog box. You need to create a new case.

   When you complete the Policy 2 tab in the Case dialog box, you will find that USAHealth Hospitalization is not one of the choices on the drop-down list of insurance carriers in the database. To complete the Policy 2 tab, you first need to add USAHealth Hospitalization to MediSoft's list of insurers.

   Select Insurance Carriers from the Lists menu. Click the New button. Complete the three tabs in the Insurance Carrier dialog box using the following information:

   Address Tab
   Code: 17
   Name: USAHealth Hospitalization
   Street: 1000 Center Street
   City: Columbus
   State: OH
   ZIP Code: 60020
   Phone: 614-022-1000
   Practice ID: 36749FG

   Options Tab
   Plan Name: USAHealth Hospitalization
   Type: Other
   Procedure Code Set: 1
   Diagnosis Code Set: 1
   Signature on File: Signature on file
   Default Billing Method: Electronic
   Print PINS on Forms: Leave blank

   EMC, Codes Tab
   EMC Receiver: 0000 National Data Corporation
   EMC Payor Number: 36740
   EMC Sub ID: 09
   NDC Record Code: 01

   Now that USAHealth Hospitalization has been added to the database, you can complete the Policy 2 tab for Stewart Robertson. Key Ø in the Insurance Coverage Percents by Service Classification box, since this policy pays a flat amount per day of hospitalization, not a percentage.

2. Make the appointment.

Part Two - December 13, 2003

MediSoft Program Date: December 13, 2003
Windows System Date: December 13, 2003

1. Print a superbill that will be used for the December 13 appointment. Circle Procedures 99203 and 93000.

2. Use the Transaction Entry dialog box to enter the charges and payments for Stewart Robertson's visit. Because he has still not reached his deductible, he pays the total charges with Check 1201.

3. Print a walkout receipt for Mr. Robertson.

Part Three - December 22, 2003

MediSoft Program Date: December 22, 2003
Windows System Date: December 22, 2003

1. Read the following account of Stewart Robertson's visit to the FCC on December 22, 2003.

   While driving to his son's soccer game, Mr. Robertson had a minor automobile accident in Jefferson and has a cut on his eyelid. He has come in to see Dr. McGrath on an emergency basis. Dr. McGrath determines that there has been no serious damage. After an examination using a local anesthetic, Dr. McGrath stitches the cut and tells Mr. Robertson to come back in a week. The procedure is simple suture with local anesthesia. Because he still has not met his deductible, Mr. Robertson pays the bill in full with Check 1220.

2. Enter all the information pertaining to this visit using the appropriate MediSoft operations.

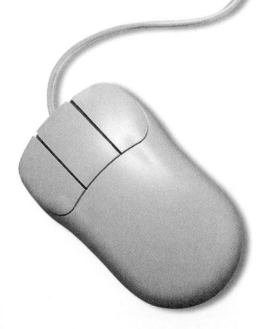

15 Printing Statements and Creating Claims

WHAT YOU NEED TO KNOW

To complete the simulations in this chapter, you need to know how to:

◆ Print patient statements.

◆ Create insurance claims.

◆ Print insurance claim forms.

Different medical practices have different billing procedures. The Family Care Center's general billing policy requires that patients pay the uninsured portion of a bill at the time service is rendered. The center bills the insurance company for the remainder. However, many exceptions are made, and bills for unpaid balances are mailed out on the fifteenth of the month for patients whose last names begin with A–L and on the thirtieth of the month for patients whose last names begin with M–Z.

SIMULATION 15-1: PRINTING PATIENT STATEMENTS

Today's date is December 22, 2003. You need to print a statement for Stewart Robertson (Simulation 14-7) so that he can take it with him.

MediSoft Program Date: December 22, 2003
Windows System Date: December 22, 2003

1. Click Patient Statements on the Reports menu.

2. Click Patient Statement in the Open Report dialog box.

3. Click the appropriate radio button to preview the statement on-screen. Click the Start button.

4. Enter Mr. Robertson's chart number in both Chart Number Range boxes.

5. Enter December 22, 2003 in both Date From Range boxes. Leave the other data selection boxes blank.

6. Click the OK button.

7. Print the statement.

8. Close the Preview Report window.

SIMULATION 15-2: CREATING INSURANCE CLAIMS

Create insurance claims for patients who have had transactions from November 14, 2003 to November 30, 2003.

MediSoft Program Date: November 30, 2003
Windows System Date: November 30, 2003

1. Click Claim Management on the Activities menu.

2. Click the Create Claims button.

3. Key *11142003* in the first Transaction Dates box and *11302003* in the second.

4. Leave the rest of the boxes blank.

5. Click the Create button.

6. Do not exit the Claim Management dialog box.

SIMULATION 15-3: PRINTING INSURANCE CLAIM FORMS

Print an insurance claim form for Carlos Lopez.

MediSoft Program Date: November 30, 2003
Windows System Date: November 30, 2003

1. In the Claim Management dialog box, select Lopez's claim.
2. Click the Print/Send button.
3. Select claims with a default billing method of paper.
4. Click the OK button.
5. Select HCFA-1500 (Primary) from the list of reports in the Open Report dialog box. Click the OK button.
6. Select the option to preview the form on-screen. Click the Start button.
7. In both the Chart Number Range boxes, enter Lopez's chart number.
8. Click the OK button.
9. Preview the form on-screen, and then print it.
10. Close the Preview Report window.

SIMULATION 15-4: PRINTING STATEMENTS FOR PATIENTS WITH OUTSTANDING BALANCES

MediSoft Program Date: November 30, 2003
Windows System Date: November 30, 2003

1. Print standard statements for all patients whose last names begin with the letters A through L and who have outstanding balances as of November 30, 2003. Figure 15-1 shows the Data Selection Questions dialog box for this task.

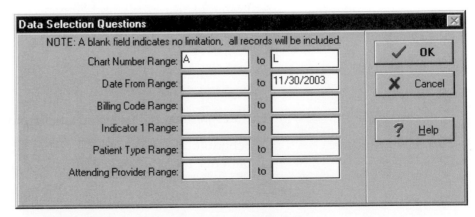

Figure 15-1 Data Selection Questions dialog box.

SIMULATION 15-5: VIEWING CLAIMS FOR PATIENTS WITH U.S. LIFE AS THEIR PRIMARY INSURANCE CARRIER

MediSoft Program Date: November 30, 2003
Windows System Date: November 30, 2003

1. Display insurance claims for all patients who have U.S. Life as their primary insurance carrier. Figure 15-2 shows the List Only Claims That Match dialog box for this task.

2. Use the Edit feature to review the transaction information contained in this claim.

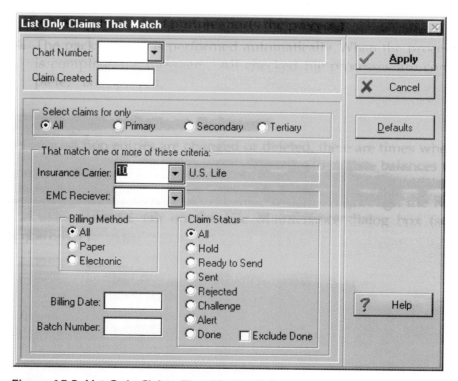

Figure 15-2 List Only Claims That Match dialog box.

SIMULATION 15-6: PUTTING IT ALL TOGETHER

For this simulation, you need to use almost all the skills you have practiced in the preceding material.

1. Enter January 5, 2004, as the program date in MediSoft.

2. Schedule appointments for January 5, 2004, for the following patients. Make sure they are scheduled for the right doctors.

Jackson, Luther	ECG, 30 minutes	9:00 a.m.
Hsu, Diane	Tine test, 15 minutes	9:00 a.m.

Hsu, Edwin	Tine test, 15 minutes	9:15 a.m.
Simmons, Jill	Strep test, quick, 15 minutes	9:00 a.m.
Arlen, Susan	Established patient, comprehensive, 1 hour	9:15 a.m.
Syzmanski, Debra	Established patient, problem focused, 30 minutes	9:30 a.m.
Giles, Sheila	Injection, 15 minutes	10:15 a.m.
Roberston, Stewart	Established patient, minimal, 15 minutes	10:30 a.m.
Battistuta, Pauline	Established patient, minimal, 15 minutes	9:30 a.m.

3. Switch the appointment times for Giles and Robertson.

4. Cancel both of the Hsus' appointments.

5. Print the appointment lists for January 5, 2004, for the three doctors.

6. Print superbills for all the appointments for the day.

7. Create new cases for all patients with appointments on January 5. Fill in the Personal and Diagnosis tabs using the following information:

Luther Jackson
Personal tab - Description box: Chest pain
Diagnosis tab - Diagnosis box: Patient's fear unfounded

Jill Simmons
Personal tab - Description box: Sore throat
Diagnosis tab - Diagnosis box: Strep throat

Susan Arlen
Personal tab - Description box: Physical examination
Diagnosis tab - Diagnosis box: Physical examination

Debra Syzmanski
Personal tab - Description box: Physical examination
Diagnosis tab - Diagnosis box: Physical examination

Sheila Giles
Personal tab - Description box: Immunization
Diagnosis tab - Diagnosis box: Immunization against tetanus

Stewart Roberston
Personal tab - Description box: Upper-respiratory infection
Diagnosis tab - Diagnosis box: Upper-respiratory infection

Pauline Battistuta
Personal tab - Description box: Carpal tunnel syndrome
Diagnosis tab - Diagnosis box: Carpal tunnel syndrome

8. Record the charge and payment transactions for each of the patients who had appointments. Jackson, Simmons, and Arlen pay their portion of the charges. Jackson pays with Check 1291, Simmons pays with check #692, and Arlen pays with Check 1022. Print walkout receipts for Jackson, Simmons, and Arlen. None of the other patients pay.

Be sure to save each one of these transactions before you proceed to the next one.

Use the Search feature in the Procedure/Payment/Adjustment List dialog box to find the correct procedure codes, or print the custom report entitled "Procedure Code List" to obtain a list of all the codes in Family Care Center's database.

You also need the following information:

Susan Arlen should be charged for these tests:
ECG
HDL cholesterol
Urine culture and colony count
Manual differential WBC

Pauline Battistuta should be charged for these X rays:
Elbow X ray
Wrist X ray
Forearm X ray

9. Print patient day sheets for all the patients with transactions on January 5, 2004.

10. Print patient statements for all patients who had appointments on January 5, 2004.

11. Create insurance claims for the day's transactions.

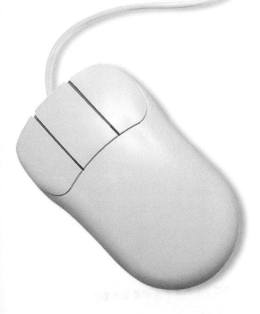

16 Filing Electronic Media Claims

WHAT YOU NEED TO KNOW

To complete the simulations in this chapter, you need to know how to:

◆ Create electronic claims.

◆ Send claims electronically to insurance carriers.

◆ Review an audit/edit report.

◆ Review claims for errors and omissions.

ELECTRONIC CLAIM REQUIREMENTS

As stated in Chapter 2, insurance carriers use different claim formats when processing electronic claims. For this reason, many medical offices send their electronic claims to a clearinghouse, which checks the data and translates it into the appropriate format for the particular carrier. The clearinghouse then sends the claim to the insurance carrier.

As the largest processor of health insurance claims in the United States, Medicare is also the industry's leader in processing electronic claims. More than 75 percent of Medicare Part B claims are processed electronically. In the near future, all Medicare- and Medicaid-participating providers may be required to submit their claims electronically.

Medicare requires that certain boxes be filled in on electronic claims. These are known as mandatory boxes. Other boxes are conditional; that is, whether they need to be filled in depends upon other information. For example, the name of a patient's employer is a conditional box; it needs to be completed only if a patient is employed. The following table lists each box that must be filled in when submitting electronic claims to Medicare and its corresponding location in MediSoft.

Table 16-1   Medicare Mandatory Boxes for Submitting Electronic Claims

Required Information	Dialog Box	Tab	Box
Insured's ID number	Case	Policy 1	Policy Number
Patient's name	Patient/Guarantor	Name, Address	Last Name First Name
Insured's policy group number	Case	Policy 1	Group Number
Patient's signature source	Patient/Guarantor	Other Information	Signature on File
Dates of service	Transaction Entry	Charge	Dates
Place of service	Transaction Entry	Charge	POS
Procedures	Transaction Entry	Charge	Procedure
Charges	Transaction Entry	Charge	Amount
Units of service	Transaction Entry	Charge	Units
Provider's signature indicator	Provider	Address	Signature on File
Provider's billing name and address	Provider	Address	Last Name First Name
Payer organization	Practice Information		Practice Name
Provider Medicare Number	Provider	PINs and IDs	PIN Medicare
Provider's pay to address	Provider	Address	Street
Provider's pay to city	Provider	Address	City
Provider's pay to state	Provider	Address	State
Provider's pay to ZIP Code	Provider	Address	Zip Code
Provider's pay to phone number	Provider	Address	Phone

SIMULATION 16-1: PERFORMING AN ON-SCREEN EDIT CHECK

Anthony Battistuta was seen by Dr. McGrath on November 14, 2003. Several charges have been entered, and an insurance claim has been created. Using the Medicare mandatory box guidelines, check to be certain that all the mandatory boxes are complete for the transactions on this claim. Make a list of any required boxes that are not complete.

SIMULATION 16-2: PREPARING A CLAIM FOR ELECTRONIC TRANSMISSION

Once data has been checked for accuracy and completeness, a claim is ready to be transmitted to the clearinghouse. While it is not possible to actually send claims in this simulation, they can be prepared for transmission. Perform all the steps necessary to submit Mr. Battistuta's claim for electronic transmission to a clearinghouse. electronic claims. When the Send Electronic Claims dialog box is displayed, do not click the Send Claims Now button. Because you are in a school setting and are not set up to submit electronic claims, click the Close button.

Source Documents

FAMILY CARE CENTER PATIENT INFORMATION FORM

*(PLEASE COMPLETE **ALL** INFORMATION)*

PATIENT'S NAME <u>Tanaka   Hiro</u>   DATE OF BIRTH <u>02</u>/<u>20</u>/<u>75</u>   SEX M ☐ F ☒   AGE <u>28</u>

      Last Name   First Name   Middle Initial   M   D   Y

PATIENT'S STATUS   Single ☒   Married ☐   Widowed ☐   Divorced ☐   Separated ☐

PATIENT'S ADDRESS (No., Street) <u>80 Cedar Lane</u>

                            City <u>Stephenson</u>   State <u>OH</u>   ZIP Code <u>60089</u>

HOME TELEPHONE (<u>614</u>) <u>555-7373</u>   SOCIAL SECURITY NUMBER   <u>812</u>   <u>73</u>   <u>6000</u>

PATIENT'S RELATIONSHIP TO INSURED   Self ☒   Spouse ☐   Child ☐   Other ☐

ALLERGIES <u>penicillin</u>   REASON FOR VISIT <u>Accident - back pain</u>

REFERRED BY <u>Dr. Bertram Brown</u>

STUDENT STATUS   Full time ☐   Part time ☐   Non-student ☒

PATIENT'S OCCUPATION <u>accountant</u>   SPOUSE'S OR PARENT'S NAME _____

EMPLOYMENT STATUS <u>full-time</u>   OCCUPATION _____

EMPLOYER'S NAME <u>McCray Manufacturing Inc</u>   EMPLOYER'S NAME _____

BUSINESS ADDRESS <u>1311 Kings Highway</u>   BUSINESS ADDRESS _____

City <u>Stephenson</u>   State <u>OH</u>   City _____ State _____

ZIP Code <u>60089</u>   ZIP Code _____

BUSINESS TELEPHONE <u>(614) 555-0000</u>   BUSINESS TELEPHONE _____
(Include Area Code)   (Include Area Code)

PRIMARY INSURANCE PLAN		IS THERE A SECONDARY HEALTH BENEFIT PLAN?

PLAN NAME	PATIENT'S ID #
Physician Alliance of Ohio	321214

POLICYHOLDER'S NAME (Last Name, First Name, Middle Initial)
Tanaka, Hiro

POLICYHOLDER'S ADDRESS (No. Street)
same as above

CITY	STATE	ZIP CODE

% OF COVERAGE	TELEPHONE (INCLUDE AREA CODE)
90	( )

POLICYHOLDER'S GROUP AND SOCIAL SECURITY NUMBER
HJ31   812-73-6000

POLICYHOLDER'S DATE OF BIRTH   SEX
2 | 20 | 75   M ☐   F ☒
M   D   Y

IS THERE A SECONDARY HEALTH BENEFIT PLAN?
☐ YES   ☒ NO   *If yes, complete below.*

OTHER POLICYHOLDER'S NAME (Last Name, First Name, Middle Initial)

EMPLOYER'S NAME OR SCHOOL NAME

INSURANCE PLAN NAME OR PROGRAM NAME

SECOND POLICY'S GROUP NUMBER AND I.D. NUMBER

POLICYHOLDER'S DATE OF BIRTH   SEX
M | D | Y   M ☐   F ☐

I/we authorize the release of the above patient's medical records for billing purposes.
Hiro Tanaka   8/9/03
    Signature   Signature   Date

I/we authorize payment of medical benefits to the physician listed below.
Hiro Tanaka   *Dr. Katherine Yan*   8/9/03
    Signature   Signature   Physician   Date

FAMILY CARE CENTER PATIENT INFORMATION FORM
*(PLEASE COMPLETE **ALL** INFORMATION)*

PATIENT'S NAME _Ramos   Juanita_   DATE OF BIRTH _4_ / _15_ / _61_   SEX M ❑ F ☒   AGE _41_
       Last Name   First Name   Middle Initial   M   D   Y

PATIENT'S STATUS   Single ☒   Married ❑   Widowed ❑   Divorced ❑   Separated ❑

PATIENT'S ADDRESS (No., Street) _75 Central Street_

                  City _Stephenson_   State _OH_   ZIP Code _60089_

HOME TELEPHONE (_614_) _888-0077_   SOCIAL SECURITY NUMBER _433_   _11_   _2710_

PATIENT'S RELATIONSHIP TO INSURED   Self ☒   Spouse ❑   Child ❑   Other ❑

ALLERGIES _____   REASON FOR VISIT _sore, red throat_

REFERRED BY _Dr. Janet Wood_

STUDENT STATUS   Full time ❑   Part time ❑   Non-student ☒

PATIENT'S OCCUPATION _supervisor_   SPOUSE'S OR PARENT'S NAME _____

EMPLOYMENT STATUS _full-time_   OCCUPATION _____

EMPLOYER'S NAME _Federal Printing School_   EMPLOYER'S NAME _____

BUSINESS ADDRESS _____   BUSINESS ADDRESS _____

City _____ State _____   City _____ State _____

ZIP Code _____   ZIP Code _____

BUSINESS TELEPHONE _(614) 555-1222_   BUSINESS TELEPHONE _____
   (Include Area Code)   (Include Area Code)

PRIMARY INSURANCE PLAN		
PLAN NAME _Champus_	PATIENT'S ID # _3021_	
POLICYHOLDER'S NAME (Last Name, First Name, Middle Initial) _Ramos, Juanita_		
POLICYHOLDER'S ADDRESS (No. Street) _same as above_		
CITY	STATE	ZIP CODE
% OF COVERAGE _100_	TELEPHONE (INCLUDE AREA CODE) ( )	
POLICYHOLDER'S GROUP AND SOCIAL SECURITY NUMBER _JOP-135_ _433-11-2710_		
POLICYHOLDER'S DATE OF BIRTH _4_ | _15_ | _61_ M ❑ F ☒		

IS THERE A SECONDARY HEALTH BENEFIT PLAN?
❑ YES   ☒ NO   *If yes, complete below.*
OTHER POLICYHOLDER'S NAME (Last Name, First Name, Middle Initial)
EMPLOYER'S NAME OR SCHOOL NAME
INSURANCE PLAN NAME OR PROGRAM NAME
SECOND POLICY'S GROUP NUMBER AND I.D. NUMBER
POLICYHOLDER'S DATE OF BIRTH   SEX   M ❑   F ❑

Regardless of any insurance coverage I/we may or may not have, it is my/our responsibility to pay the entire bill. In the event that this office needs to obtain legal assistance in collection of any unpaid balance, I/we agree to pay costs and attorney fees, as allowable by law, and acknowledge receipt of a photocopy of this agreement.

I/we authorize the release of the above patient's medical records for billing purposes.

Juanita Ramos   _2/10/03_
    Signature   Signature   Date

I/we authorize payment of medical benefits to the physician listed below.

Juanita Ramos   _Dr. Jessica Rudner_   _2/10/03_
    Signature   Signature   Physician   Date

Physician's Notes for Hiro Tanaka

Condition related to an auto accident that occurred in Stephenson, Ohio, on August 8, 2003.

Doctor visit, August 9, 2003.

Patient disabled from August 9, 2003 to October 1, 2003.

Was hospitalized from August 9, 2003 to August 15, 2003.

Partially disabled from October 1 to November 15, 2003.

Unable to work August 9, 2003 to November 15, 2003.

Death Status: Able to carry on normal activity.

Family Care Center
285 Stephenson Boulevard
Stephenson, OH 60089
(614)555-0000

Date: 8/9/03

Name **Hiro Tanaka**

Chart Number **TANAKHIØ**

Physician **Dr. Katherine Yan**

01	patient payment, cash	85651	erythrocyte sedimentation rate--non-auto
02	patient payment, check	86403	strep test, quick
03	insurance carrier payment	86585	tuberculosis, tine test
04	insurance company adjustment	86588	direct streptococcus screen
05	adjustment, patient	87072	culture by commercial kit, nonurine...
06	OhioCare HMO Charge - $10	87076	bacterial culture, anerobic, with GC...
07	OhioCare HMO Charge - $15	87086	urine culture and colony count
12011	simple suture--face--local anes.	90703	tetanus injection
29125	application of short arm splint; static	90782	injection with material, subcutaneous or
29425	application of short leg cast, walking	92516	facial nerve function studies
45378	colonoscopy--diagnostic	93000	Electrocardiogram--ECG with interpret...
45380	colonoscopy--with biopsy	93015	Treadmill stress test, with physician...
50390	aspiration of renal cyst by needle	96900	ultraviolet light treatment
71010	chest x-ray, single view, frontal	99070	supplies and materials provided
71020	chest x-ray, two views, frontal & lat...	99201	OF--new patient, problem focused
71030	chest x-ray, complete, four views	99202	OF--new patient, expanded
73070	elbow x-ray, AP and lateral views	99203	OF--new patient, detailed history and...
73090	forearm x-ray, AP and lateral views	99204	OF--new patient, comprehensive history..
73100	wrist x-ray, AP and lateral views	99205	OF--new patient, comprehensive history..
73510	hip x-ray, complete, two views	99211	OF--established patient, minimal
73600	ankle x-ray, AP and lateral views	99212	OF--established patient, problem focused
80019	19 clinical chemistry tests	99213	OF--established patient, expanded
80061	lipid panel	99214	OF--established patient, detailed...
82270	blood screening, occult; feces	99215	OF--established patient, comprehensive..
82947	glucose screening--quantitative	99394	established patient, adolescent, per...
82951	glucose tolerance test, three specimens	99396	established patient, 40-64 years, per...
83718	HDL cholesterol		
84478	triglycerides test		
85007	manual differential WBC		
85022	hemogram, automated, and manual...		

Payments

Diagnosis 724.2

Remarks

Family Care Center
285 Stephenson Boulevard
Stephenson, OH 60089
(614)555-0000

Date: 2/10/03

Name Juanita Ramos

Chart Number RAMOSJU0

Physician Dr. Jessica Rudner

01	patient payment, cash		85651	erythrocyte sedimentation rate--non-auto
02	patient payment, check		86403	strep test, quick
03	insurance carrier payment		86585	tuberculosis, tine test
04	insurance company adjustment		86588	direct streptococcus screen
05	adjustment, patient		87072	culture by commercial kit, nonurine...
06	OhioCare HMO Charge - $10		87076	bacterial culture, anerobic, with GC...
07	OhioCare HMO Charge - $15		87086	urine culture and colony count
12011	simple suture--face--local anes.		90703	tetanus injection
29125	application of short arm splint; static		90782	injection with material, subcutaneous or
29425	application of short leg cast, walking		92516	facial nerve function studies
45378	colonoscopy--diagnostic		93000	Electrocardiogram--ECG with interpret...
45380	colonoscopy--with biopsy		93015	Treadmill stress test, with physician...
50390	aspiration of renal cyst by needle		96900	ultraviolet light treatment
71010	chest x-ray, single view, frontal		99070	supplies and materials provided
71020	chest x-ray, two views, frontal & lat...		99201	OF--new patient, problem focused
71030	chest x-ray, complete, four views		99202	OF--new patient, expanded
73070	elbow x-ray, AP and lateral views		99203	OF--new patient, detailed history and...
73090	forearm x-ray, AP and lateral views		99204	OF--new patient, comprehensive history..
73100	wrist x-ray, AP and lateral views		99205	OF--new patient, comprehensive history..
73510	hip x-ray, complete, two views		99211	OF--established patient, minimal
73600	ankle x-ray, AP and lateral views		99212	OF--established patient, problem focused
80019	19 clinical chemistry tests		99213	OF--established patient, expanded
80061	lipid panel		99214	OF--established patient, detailed...
82270	blood screening, occult; feces		99215	OF--established patient, comprehensive..
82947	glucose screening--quantitative		99394	established patient, adolescent, per...
82951	glucose tolerance test, three specimens		99396	established patient, 40-64 years, per...
83718	HDL cholesterol			
84478	triglycerides test			
85007	manual differential WBC			
85022	hemogram, automated, and manual...			

Payments _____

Diagnosis 034.0

Remarks _____

Family Care Center
285 Stephenson Boulevard
Stephenson, OH 60089
(614)555-0000

Date: 12/8/03

Chart Number JONESL0

Name Elizabeth Jones

Physician Dr. Katherine Yan

01	patient payment, cash	85651	erythrocyte sedimentation rate--non-auto
02	patient payment, check	86403	strep test, quick
03	insurance carrier payment	86585	tuberculosis, tine test
04	insurance company adjustment	86588	direct streptococcus screen
05	adjustment, patient	87072	culture by commercial kit, nonurine...
06	OhioCare HMO Charge - $10	87076	bacterial culture, anerobic, with GC...
07	OhioCare HMO Charge - $15	87086	urine culture and colony count
12011	simple suture--face--local anes.	90703	tetanus injection
29125	application of short arm splint; static	90782	injection with material, subcutaneous or
29425	application of short leg cast, walking	92516	facial nerve function studies
45378	colonoscopy--diagnostic	93000	Electrocardiogram--ECG with interpret...
45380	colonoscopy--with biopsy	93015	Treadmill stress test, with physician...
50390	aspiration of renal cyst by needle	96900	ultraviolet light treatment
71010	chest x-ray, single view, frontal	99070	supplies and materials provided
71020	chest x-ray, two views, frontal & lat...	99201	OF--new patient, problem focused
71030	chest x-ray, complete, four views	99202	OF--new patient, expanded
73070	elbow x-ray, AP and lateral views	99203	OF--new patient, detailed history and...
73090	forearm x-ray, AP and lateral views	99204	OF--new patient, comprehensive history..
73100	wrist x-ray, AP and lateral views	99205	OF--new patient, comprehensive history..
73510	hip x-ray, complete, two views	99211	OF--established patient, minimal
73600	ankle x-ray, AP and lateral views	99212	OF--established patient, problem focused
80019	19 clinical chemistry tests	(99213)	OF--established patient, expanded
80061	lipid panel	99214	OF--established patient, detailed...
82270	blood screening, occult; feces	99215	OF--established patient, comprehensive..
82947	glucose screening--quantitative	99394	established patient, adolescent, per...
82951	glucose tolerance test, three specimens	99396	established patient, 40-64 years, per...
83718	HDL cholesterol		
84478	triglycerides test		
85007	manual differential WBC		
85022	hemogram, automated, and manual...		

Payments _____

Diagnosis 250.0

Remarks _____

Family Care Center
285 Stephenson Boulevard
Stephenson, OH 60089
(614)555-0000

Date: 12/8/03

Name **John Fitzwilliams**

Chart Number **FITZWJO0**

Physician **Dr. John Rudner**

01	patient payment, cash	85651	erythrocyte sedimentation rate--non-auto
02	patient payment, check	86403	strep test, quick
03	insurance carrier payment	86585	tuberculosis, tine test
04	insurance company adjustment	86588	direct streptococcus screen
05	adjustment, patient	87072	culture by commercial kit, nonurine...
06	OhioCare HMO Charge - $10	87076	bacterial culture, anerobic, with GC...
07	OhioCare HMO Charge - $15	87086	urine culture and colony count
12011	simple suture--face--local anes.	90703	tetanus injection
29125	application of short arm splint; static	90782	injection with material, subcutaneous or
29425	application of short leg cast, walking	92516	facial nerve function studies
45378	colonoscopy--diagnostic	93000	Electrocardiogram--ECG with interpret...
45380	colonoscopy--with biopsy	93015	Treadmill stress test, with physician...
50390	aspiration of renal cyst by needle	96900	ultraviolet light treatment
71010	chest x-ray, single view, frontal	99070	supplies and materials provided
71020	chest x-ray, two views, frontal & lat...	99201	OF--new patient, problem focused
71030	chest x-ray, complete, four views	99202	OF--new patient, expanded
73070	elbow x-ray, AP and lateral views	99203	OF--new patient, detailed history and...
73090	forearm x-ray, AP and lateral views	99204	OF--new patient, comprehensive history..
73100	wrist x-ray, AP and lateral views	99205	OF--new patient, comprehensive history..
73510	hip x-ray, complete, two views	99211	OF--established patient, minimal
73600	ankle x-ray, AP and lateral views	99212	OF--established patient, problem focused
80019	19 clinical chemistry tests	99213	OF--established patient, expanded
80061	lipid panel	99214	OF--established patient, detailed...
82270	blood screening, occult; feces	99215	OF--established patient, comprehensive..
82947	glucose screening--quantitative	99394	established patient, adolescent, per...
82951	glucose tolerance test, three specimens	99396	established patient, 40-64 years, per...
83718	HDL cholesterol		
84478	triglycerides test		
85007	manual differential WBC		
85022	hemogram, automated, and manual...		

Payments _____

Diagnosis **531.30**

Remarks _____

_____

Family Care Center
285 Stephenson Boulevard
Stephenson, OH 60089
(614)555-0000

Date: 11/14/03

Name Anthony Battistuta

Chart Number BATTIAN0

Physician Dr. McGrath

01	patient payment, cash	85651	erythrocyte sedimentation rate--non-auto
02	patient payment, check	86403	strep test, quick
03	insurance carrier payment	86585	tuberculosis, tine test
04	insurance company adjustment	86588	direct streptococcus screen
05	adjustment, patient	87072	culture by commercial kit, nonurine...
06	OhioCare HMO Charge - $10	87076	bacterial culture, anerobic, with GC...
07	OhioCare HMO Charge - $15	(87086	urine culture and colony count)
12011	simple suture--face--local anes.	90703	tetanus injection
29125	application of short arm splint; static	90782	injection with material, subcutaneous or
29425	application of short leg cast, walking	92516	facial nerve function studies
45378	colonoscopy--diagnostic	93000	Electrocardiogram--ECG with interpret...
45380	colonoscopy--with biopsy	93015	Treadmill stress test, with physician...
50390	aspiration of renal cyst by needle	96900	ultraviolet light treatment
71010	chest x-ray, single view, frontal	99070	supplies and materials provided
71020	chest x-ray, two views, frontal & lat...	99201	OF--new patient, problem focused
71030	chest x-ray, complete, four views	99202	OF--new patient, expanded
73070	elbow x-ray, AP and lateral views	99203	OF--new patient, detailed history and...
73090	forearm x-ray, AP and lateral views	99204	OF--new patient, comprehensive history..
73100	wrist x-ray, AP and lateral views	99205	OF--new patient, comprehensive history..
73510	hip x-ray, complete, two views	99211	OF--established patient, minimal
73600	ankle x-ray, AP and lateral views	(99212	OF--established patient, problem focused)
80019	19 clinical chemistry tests	99213	OF--established patient, expanded
80061	lipid panel	99214	OF--established patient, detailed...
82270	blood screening, occult; feces	99215	OF--established patient, comprehensive..
82947	glucose screening--quantitative	99394	established patient, adolescent, per...
(82951	glucose tolerance test, three specimens) $40	99396	established patient, 40-64 years, per...
83718	HDL cholesterol		
84478	triglycerides test		
85007	manual differential WBC		
85022	hemogram, automated, and manual...		

Payments _____

Diagnosis diabetes

Remarks New address:

36 Grant Blvd.

Grandville, OH 60092

(614)029-3333

Family Care Center
285 Stephenson Boulevard
Stephenson, OH 60089
(614)555-0000

Date: 11/14/03   **Name** **Lawana Brooks**

Chart Number **BROOKSLA0**   **Physician** **Dr. McGrath**

01	patient payment, cash	85651	erythrocyte sedimentation rate--non-auto
02	patient payment, check	86403	strep test, quick
03	insurance carrier payment	86585	tuberculosis, tine test
04	insurance company adjustment	86588	direct streptococcus screen
05	adjustment, patient	87072	culture by commercial kit, nonurine...
06	OhioCare HMO Charge - $10	87076	bacterial culture, anerobic, with GC...
07	OhioCare HMO Charge - $15	87086	urine culture and colony count
12011	simple suture--face--local anes.	90703	tetanus injection
(29125)	application of short arm splint; static	90782	injection with material, subcutaneous or
29425	application of short leg cast, walking	92516	facial nerve function studies
45378	colonoscopy--diagnostic	93000	Electrocardiogram--ECG with interpret...
45380	colonoscopy--with biopsy	93015	Treadmill stress test, with physician...
50390	aspiration of renal cyst by needle	96900	ultraviolet light treatment
71010	chest x-ray, single view, frontal	99070	supplies and materials provided
71020	chest x-ray, two views, frontal & lat...	99201	OF--new patient, problem focused
71030	chest x-ray, complete, four views	99202	OF--new patient, expanded
73070	elbow x-ray, AP and lateral views	99203	OF--new patient, detailed history and...
(73090)	forearm x-ray, AP and lateral views	99204	OF--new patient, comprehensive history..
73100	wrist x-ray, AP and lateral views	99205	OF--new patient, comprehensive history..
73510	hip x-ray, complete, two views	99211	OF--established patient, minimal
73600	ankle x-ray, AP and lateral views	(99212)	OF--established patient, problem focused **$100**
80019	19 clinical chemistry tests	99213	OF--established patient, expanded
80061	lipid panel	99214	OF--established patient, detailed...
82270	blood screening, occult; feces	99215	OF--established patient, comprehensive..
82947	glucose screening--quantitative	99394	established patient, adolescent, per...
82951	glucose tolerance test, three specimens	99396	established patient, 40-64 years, per...
83718	HDL cholesterol		
84478	triglycerides test		
85007	manual differential WBC		
85022	hemogram, automated, and manual...		

Payments _____   **Remarks** Slipped on coffee spill on floor and injured arm

Diagnosis 841.0 / E885 / E849.3

Family Care Center
285 Stephenson Boulevard
Stephenson, OH 60089
(614)555-0000

Date: 11/14/03

Chart Number HSUEDWIØ

Name Edwin Hsu

Physician Dr. McGrath

01	patient payment, cash	85651	erythrocyte sedimentation rate--non-auto
02	patient payment, check	86403	strep test, quick
03	insurance carrier payment	86585	tuberculosis, tine test
04	insurance company adjustment	86588	direct streptococcus screen
05	adjustment, patient	87072	culture by commercial kit, nonurine...
06	OhioCare HMO Charge - $10	87076	bacterial culture, anerobic, with GC...
07	OhioCare HMO Charge - $15	87086	urine culture and colony count
12011	simple suture--face--local anes.	90703	tetanus injection
29125	application of short arm splint; static	90782	injection with material, subcutaneous or
29425	application of short leg cast, walking	92516	facial nerve function studies
45378	colonoscopy--diagnostic	93000	Electrocardiogram--ECG with interpret...
45380	colonoscopy--with biopsy	93015	Treadmill stress test, with physician...
50390	aspiration of renal cyst by needle	96900	ultraviolet light treatment
71010	chest x-ray, single view, frontal	99070	supplies and materials provided
71020	chest x-ray, two views, frontal & lat...	99201	OF--new patient, problem focused
71030	chest x-ray, complete, four views	99202	OF--new patient, expanded
73070	elbow x-ray, AP and lateral views	99203	OF--new patient, detailed history and...
73090	forearm x-ray, AP and lateral views	99204	OF--new patient, comprehensive history..
73100	wrist x-ray, AP and lateral views	99205	OF--new patient, comprehensive history..
73510	hip x-ray, complete, two views	(99211)	OF--established patient, minimal
73600	ankle x-ray, AP and lateral views	99212	OF--established patient, problem focused
80019	19 clinical chemistry tests	99213	OF--established patient, expanded
80061	lipid panel	99214	OF--established patient, detailed...
82270	blood screening, occult; feces	99215	OF--established patient, comprehensive..
82947	glucose screening--quantitative	99394	established patient, adolescent, per...
82951	glucose tolerance test, three specimens	99396	established patient, 40-64 years, per...
83718	HDL cholesterol		
84478	triglycerides test		
85007	manual differential WBC		
85022	hemogram, automated, and manual...		

New insurance carrier:
Midwest Select
Policy #51249, Group #256

Payments $10 cash

Diagnosis 461.9 acute sinusitis

Remarks New address:
56 Reynolds St.
Stephenson, OH 60089
(614)022-3010

FAMILY CARE CENTER PATIENT INFORMATION FORM

(PLEASE COMPLETE ALL INFORMATION)

PATIENT'S NAME <u>Syzmanski Hannah</u> DATE OF BIRTH <u>02</u>/ <u>26</u>/ <u>88</u> SEX M ☐ F ☒ AGE <u>15</u>

       Last Name First Name Middle Initial   M   D   Y

PATIENT'S STATUS Single ☒ Married ☐ Widowed ☐ Divorced ☐ Separated ☐

PATIENT'S ADDRESS (No., Street) <u>3 Broadbrook Lane</u>

        City <u>Stephenson</u> State <u>OH</u> ZIP Code <u>60089</u>

HOME TELEPHONE (<u>614</u>) <u>086-4444</u> SOCIAL SECURITY NUMBER <u>907</u> <u>66</u> <u>0003</u>

PATIENT'S RELATIONSHIP TO INSURED Self ☐ Spouse ☐ Child ☒ Other ☐

ALLERGIES <u>bee stings</u> REASON FOR VISIT <u>physical</u>

REFERRED BY <u>Dr. Harold Gearhart</u>

STUDENT STATUS Full time ☒ Part time ☐ Non-student ☐

PATIENT'S OCCUPATION_____

EMPLOYMENT STATUS_____

EMPLOYER'S NAME _____

BUSINESS ADDRESS _____

City_____ State_____

ZIP Code _____

BUSINESS TELEPHONE _____

  (Include Area Code)

SPOUSE'S OR PARENT'S NAME_____

OCCUPATION _____

EMPLOYER'S NAME_____

BUSINESS ADDRESS_____

City _____ State_____

ZIP Code _____

BUSINESS TELEPHONE_____

  (Include Area Code)

PRIMARY INSURANCE PLAN	
PLAN NAME	PATIENT'S ID #
POLICYHOLDER'S NAME (Last Name, First Name, Middle Initial)	
POLICYHOLDER'S ADDRESS (No. Street)	

CITY	STATE	ZIP CODE
% OF COVERAGE	TELEPHONE (INCLUDE AREA CODE) ( )	

POLICYHOLDER'S GROUP AND SOCIAL SECURITY NUMBER

POLICYHOLDER'S DATE OF BIRTH SEX
M D Y M ☐ F ☒

IS THERE A SECONDARY HEALTH BENEFIT PLAN?

☐ YES ☐ NO If yes, complete below.

OTHER POLICYHOLDER'S NAME (Last Name, First Name, Middle Initial)

EMPLOYER'S NAME OR SCHOOL NAME

INSURANCE PLAN NAME OR PROGRAM NAME

SECOND POLICY'S GROUP NUMBER AND I.D. NUMBER

POLICYHOLDER'S DATE OF BIRTH SEX
M D Y M ☐ F ☐

Regardless of any insurance coverage I/we may or may not have, it is my/our responsibility to pay the entire bill. In the event that this office needs to obtain legal assistance in collection of any unpaid balance, I/we agree to pay costs and attorney fees, as allowable by law, and acknowledge receipt of a photocopy of this agreement.

I/we authorize the release of the above patient's medical records for billing purposes.

<u>Debra Syzmanski</u> _____ <u>11/14/03</u>
   Signature   Signature   Date

I/we authorize payment of medical benefits to the physician listed below.

<u>Debra Syzmanski</u> _____ <u>Dr. Dana Banu</u> <u>11/14/03</u>
   Signature   Signature   Physician   Date

```
┌─────────────────────────────┐
│      Family Care Center     │
│   285 Stephenson Boulevard   │
│     Stephenson, OH 60089     │
│        (614)555-0000         │
└─────────────────────────────┘
```

Date: 11/14/03

Name Hannah Syzmanski

Chart Number SYZMAHA0

Physician Dr. Banu

01	patient payment, cash	85651	erythrocyte sedimentation rate--non-auto
02	patient payment, check	86403	strep test, quick
03	insurance carrier payment	86585	tuberculosis, tine test
04	insurance company adjustment	86588	direct streptococcus screen
05	adjustment, patient	87072	culture by commercial kit, nonurine...
06	OhioCare HMO Charge - $10	87076	bacterial culture, anaerobic, with GC...
07	OhioCare HMO Charge - $15	87086	urine culture and colony count
12011	simple suture--face--local anes.	90703	tetanus injection
29125	application of short arm splint; static	90782	injection with material, subcutaneous or
29425	application of short leg cast, walking	92516	facial nerve function studies
45378	colonoscopy--diagnostic	93000	Electrocardiogram--ECG with interpret...
45380	colonoscopy--with biopsy	93015	Treadmill stress test, with physician...
50390	aspiration of renal cyst by needle	96900	ultraviolet light treatment
71010	chest x-ray, single view, frontal	99070	supplies and materials provided
71020	chest x-ray, two views, frontal & lat...	99201	OF--new patient, problem focused
71030	chest x-ray, complete, four views	99202	OF--new patient, expanded
73070	elbow x-ray, AP and lateral views	(99203)	OF--new patient, detailed history and...
73090	forearm x-ray, AP and lateral views	99204	OF--new patient, comprehensive history..
73100	wrist x-ray, AP and lateral views	99205	OF--new patient, comprehensive history..
73510	hip x-ray, complete, two views	99211	OF--established patient, minimal
73600	ankle x-ray, AP and lateral views	99212	OF--established patient, problem focused
80019	19 clinical chemistry tests	99213	OF--established patient, expanded
80061	lipid panel	99214	OF--established patient, detailed...
82270	blood screening, occult; feces	99215	OF--established patient, comprehensive..
82947	glucose screening--quantitative	99394	established patient, adolescent, per...
82951	glucose tolerance test, three specimens	99396	established patient, 40-64 years, per...
83718	HDL cholesterol		
84478	triglycerides test		
85007	manual differential WBC		
85022	hemogram, automated, and manual...		

Payments _____

Remarks _____

Diagnosis V70.0 _____

287

Family Care Center
285 Stephenson Boulevard
Stephenson, OH 60089
(614)555-0000

Date: 11/17/03

Chart Number LOPEZCAØ

Name Carlos Lopez

Physician Dr. McGrath

01	patient payment, cash		85651	erythrocyte sedimentation rate--non-auto
02	patient payment, check		86403	strep test, quick
03	insurance carrier payment		86585	tuberculosis, tine test
04	insurance company adjustment		86588	direct streptococcus screen
05	adjustment, patient		87072	culture by commercial kit, nonurine...
06	OhioCare HMO Charge - $10		87076	bacterial culture, anerobic, with GC...
07	OhioCare HMO Charge - $15		87086	urine culture and colony count
12011	simple suture--face--local anes.		90703	tetanus injection
29125	application of short arm splint; static		90782	injection with material, subcutaneous or
29425	application of short leg cast, walking		92516	facial nerve function studies
45378	colonoscopy--diagnostic		93000	Electrocardiogram--ECG with interpret...
45380	colonoscopy--with biopsy		93015	Treadmill stress test, with physician...
50390	aspiration of renal cyst by needle		96900	ultraviolet light treatment
71010	chest x-ray, single view, frontal		99070	supplies and materials provided
71020	chest x-ray, two views, frontal & lat...		99201	OF--new patient, problem focused
71030	chest x-ray, complete, four views		99202	OF--new patient, expanded
73070	elbow x-ray, AP and lateral views		99203	OF--new patient, detailed history and...
73090	forearm x-ray, AP and lateral views		99204	OF--new patient, comprehensive history..
73100	wrist x-ray, AP and lateral views		99205	OF--new patient, comprehensive history..
73510	hip x-ray, complete, two views		99211	OF--established patient, minimal
73600	ankle x-ray, AP and lateral views		99212	OF--established patient, problem focused
80019	19 clinical chemistry tests		99213	OF--established patient, expanded
80061	lipid panel		99214	OF--established patient, detailed...
82270	blood screening, occult; feces		99215	OF--established patient, comprehensive..
82947	glucose screening--quantitative		99394	established patient, adolescent, per...
82951	glucose tolerance test, three specimens		99396	established patient, 40-64 years, per...
83718	HDL cholesterol			
84478	triglycerides test			
85007	manual differential WBC			
85022	hemogram, automated, and manual...			

Payments _____

Diagnosis V65.5 patient fear unfounded

Remarks Patient had palpitations

_____

FAMILY CARE CENTER PATIENT INFORMATION FORM

*(PLEASE COMPLETE **ALL** INFORMATION)*

PATIENT'S NAME _Palmer Christopher_   DATE OF BIRTH _1_ / _5_ / _48_   SEX M ☒ F ☐   AGE _55_

Last Name   First Name   Middle Initial   M   D   Y

PATIENT'S STATUS   Single ☒   Married ☐   Widowed ☐   Divorced ☐   Separated ☐

PATIENT'S ADDRESS (No., Street) _17 Red Oak Lane_

City _Jefferson_   State _OH_   ZIP Code _60093_

HOME TELEPHONE (_614_) _077-2249_   SOCIAL SECURITY NUMBER _607_ _49_ _7620_

PATIENT'S RELATIONSHIP TO INSURED   Self ☒   Spouse ☐   Child ☐   Other ☐

ALLERGIES _____   REASON FOR VISIT _trouble breathing_

REFERRED BY _Dr. Marion Davis_

STUDENT STATUS   Full time ☐   Part time ☐   Non-student ☒

PATIENT'S OCCUPATION _____   SPOUSE'S OR PARENT'S NAME _____

EMPLOYMENT STATUS _unemployed-disabled_   OCCUPATION _____

EMPLOYER'S NAME _____   EMPLOYER'S NAME _____

BUSINESS ADDRESS _____   BUSINESS ADDRESS _____

City _____ State _____   City _____ State _____

ZIP Code _____   ZIP Code _____

BUSINESS TELEPHONE _____   BUSINESS TELEPHONE _____
(Include Area Code)   (Include Area Code)

PRIMARY INSURANCE PLAN	
PLAN NAME _Medicaid_	PATIENT'S ID # _607497620_
POLICYHOLDER'S NAME (Last Name, First Name, Middle Initial) _Palmer, Christopher_	
POLICYHOLDER'S ADDRESS (No. Street) _same as above_	

CITY	STATE	ZIP CODE

% OF COVERAGE _100_	TELEPHONE (INCLUDE AREA CODE) ( )
POLICYHOLDER'S GROUP AND SOCIAL SECURITY NUMBER _607-49-7620_	
POLICYHOLDER'S DATE OF BIRTH _1_ _5_ _48_ M D Y	SEX M ☒ F ☐

IS THERE A SECONDARY HEALTH BENEFIT PLAN?
☐ YES ☒ NO   *If yes, complete below.*
OTHER POLICYHOLDER'S NAME (Last Name, First Name, Middle Initial)
EMPLOYER'S NAME OR SCHOOL NAME
INSURANCE PLAN NAME OR PROGRAM NAME
SECOND POLICY'S GROUP NUMBER AND I.D. NUMBER
POLICYHOLDER'S DATE OF BIRTH   SEX M ☐ F ☐ M D Y

Regardless of any insurance coverage I/we may or may not have, it is my/our responsibility to pay the entire bill. In the event that this office needs to obtain legal assistance in collection of any unpaid balance, I/we agree to pay costs and attorney fees, as allowable by law, and acknowledge receipt of a photocopy of this agreement.

I/we authorize the release of the above patient's medical records for billing purposes.

Christopher Palmer _____   _____   _11/17/03_
Signature   Signature   Date

I/we authorize payment of medical benefits to the physician listed below.

Christopher Palmer _____   _____   _Dr. Robert Beach_   _11/17/03_
Signature   Signature   Physician   Date

```
┌─────────────────────────────┐
│      Family Care Center      │
│    285 Stephenson Boulevard  │
│      Stephenson, OH 60089    │
│        (614)555-0000         │
└─────────────────────────────┘
```

Date: 11/17/03

Chart Number PALMECH0

Name Christopher Palmer

Physician Dr. Beach

01	patient payment, cash		85651	erythrocyte sedimentation rate--non-auto
02	patient payment, check		86403	strep test, quick
03	insurance carrier payment		86585	tuberculosis, tine test
04	insurance company adjustment		86588	direct streptococcus screen
05	adjustment, patient		87072	culture by commercial kit, nonurine...
06	OhioCare HMO Charge - $10		87076	bacterial culture, anerobic, with GC...
07	OhioCare HMO Charge - $15		87086	urine culture and colony count
12011	simple suture--face--local anes.		90703	tetanus injection
29125	application of short arm splint; static		90782	injection with material, subcutaneous or
29425	application of short leg cast, walking		92516	facial nerve function studies
45378	colonoscopy--diagnostic		93000	Electrocardiogram--ECG with interpret...
45380	colonoscopy--with biopsy		93015	Treadmill stress test, with physician...
50390	aspiration of renal cyst by needle		96900	ultraviolet light treatment
71010	chest x-ray, single view, frontal		99070	supplies and materials provided
(71020)	chest x-ray, two views, frontal & lat...		(99201)	OF--new patient, problem focused
71030	chest x-ray, complete, four views		99202	OF--new patient, expanded
73070	elbow x-ray, AP and lateral views		99203	OF--new patient, detailed history and...
73090	forearm x-ray, AP and lateral views		99204	OF--new patient, comprehensive history..
73100	wrist x-ray, AP and lateral views		99205	OF--new patient, comprehensive history..
73510	hip x-ray, complete, two views		99211	OF--established patient, minimal
73600	ankle x-ray, AP and lateral views		99212	OF--established patient, problem focused
80019	19 clinical chemistry tests		99213	OF--established patient, expanded
80061	lipid panel		99214	OF--established patient, detailed...
82270	blood screening, occult; feces		99215	OF--established patient, comprehensive..
82947	glucose screening--quantitative		99394	established patient, adolescent, per...
82951	glucose tolerance test, three specimens		99396	established patient, 40-64 years, per...
83718	HDL cholesterol			
84478	triglycerides test			
85007	manual differential WBC			
85022	hemogram, automated, and manual...			

Payments _____

Diagnosis 485 bronchopneumonia

Remarks _____

Family Care Center
285 Stephenson Boulevard
Stephenson, OH 60089
(614)555-0000

Date: 11/17/03

Name Diane Hsu

Chart Number HSUDIAN0

Physician Dr. McGrath

01	patient payment, cash		85651	erythrocyte sedimentation rate--non-auto	
02	patient payment, check		86403	strep test, quick	
03	insurance carrier payment		86585	tuberculosis, tine test	
04	insurance company adjustment		86588	direct streptococcus screen	
05	adjustment, patient		87072	culture by commercial kit, nonurine...	
06	OhioCare HMO Charge - $10		87076	bacterial culture, anerobic, with GC...	
07	OhioCare HMO Charge - $15		87086	urine culture and colony count	
12011	simple suture--face--local anes.		90703	tetanus injection	
29125	application of short arm splint; static		90782	injection with material, subcutaneous or	flu shot $15
29425	application of short leg cast, walking		92516	facial nerve function studies	
45378	colonoscopy--diagnostic		93000	Electrocardiogram--ECG with interpret...	
45380	colonoscopy--with biopsy		93015	Treadmill stress test, with physician...	
50390	aspiration of renal cyst by needle		96900	ultraviolet light treatment	
71010	chest x-ray, single view, frontal		99070	supplies and materials provided	
71020	chest x-ray, two views, frontal & lat...		99201	OF--new patient, problem focused	
71030	chest x-ray, complete, four views		99202	OF--new patient, expanded	
73070	elbow x-ray, AP and lateral views		99203	OF--new patient, detailed history and...	
73090	forearm x-ray, AP and lateral views		99204	OF--new patient, comprehensive history..	
73100	wrist x-ray, AP and lateral views		99205	OF--new patient, comprehensive history..	
73510	hip x-ray, complete, two views		99211	OF--established patient, minimal	
73600	ankle x-ray, AP and lateral views		99212	OF--established patient, problem focused	
80019	19 clinical chemistry tests		99213	OF--established patient, expanded	
80061	lipid panel		99214	OF--established patient, detailed...	
82270	blood screening, occult; feces		99215	OF--established patient, comprehensive..	
82947	glucose screening--quantitative		99394	established patient, adolescent, per...	
82951	glucose tolerance test, three specimens		99396	established patient, 40-64 years, per...	
83718	HDL cholesterol				
84478	triglycerides test				
85007	manual differential WBC				
85022	hemogram, automated, and manual...				

Payments _____

Diagnosis 487.1 influenza

Remarks Next appt. 1 week from today,
2:00 p.m., 15 minutes

Family Care Center
285 Stephenson Boulevard
Stephenson, OH 60089
(614)555-0000

Date: 11/17/03

Name Michael Syzmanski

Chart Number SYZMAMIØ

Physician Dr. Banu

01	patient payment, cash		85651	erythrocyte sedimentation rate--non-auto
02	patient payment, check		86403	strep test, quick
03	insurance carrier payment		86585	tuberculosis, tine test
04	insurance company adjustment		86588	direct streptococcus screen
05	adjustment, patient		87072	culture by commercial kit, nonurine...
06	OhioCare HMO Charge - $10		87076	bacterial culture, anerobic, with GC...
07	OhioCare HMO Charge - $15		87086	urine culture and colony count
12011	simple suture--face--local anes.		90703	tetanus injection
29125	application of short arm splint; static		90782	injection with material, subcutaneous or
29425	application of short leg cast, walking		92516	facial nerve function studies
45378	colonoscopy--diagnostic		93000	Electrocardiogram--ECG with interpret...
45380	colonoscopy--with biopsy		93015	Treadmill stress test, with physician...
50390	aspiration of renal cyst by needle		96900	ultraviolet light treatment
71010	chest x-ray, single view, frontal		99070	supplies and materials provided
71020	chest x-ray, two views, frontal & lat...		99201	OF--new patient, problem focused
71030	chest x-ray, complete, four views		99202	OF--new patient, expanded
73070	elbow x-ray, AP and lateral views		99203	OF--new patient, detailed history and...
73090	forearm x-ray, AP and lateral views		99204	OF--new patient, comprehensive history..
73100	wrist x-ray, AP and lateral views		99205	OF--new patient, comprehensive history..
73510	hip x-ray, complete, two views		99211	OF--established patient, minimal
73600	ankle x-ray, AP and lateral views		99212	OF--established patient, problem focused
80019	19 clinical chemistry tests		99213	OF--established patient, expanded
80061	lipid panel		99214	OF--established patient, detailed...
82270	blood screening, occult; feces		99215	OF--established patient, comprehensive..
82947	glucose screening--quantitative		99394	established patient, adolescent, per...
82951	glucose tolerance test, three specimens		99396	established patient, 40-64 years, per...
83718	HDL cholesterol			
84478	triglycerides test			
85007	manual differential WBC			
85022	hemogram, automated, and manual...			

Outside Lab Work:
stool occult $40

Payments $34.00   Check #319

Diagnosis 455.6 hemorrhoids

Remarks Rectal bleeding -- first
experienced 11/10/03

FAMILY CARE CENTER PATIENT INFORMATION FORM

*(PLEASE COMPLETE **ALL** INFORMATION)*

PATIENT'S NAME _Robertson Stewart_ DATE OF BIRTH _12_/_21_/_63_ SEX M ☒ F ☐ AGE _39_
Last Name   First Name   Middle Initial   M   D   Y

PATIENT'S STATUS   Single ☐   Married ☐   Widowed ☐   Divorced ☒   Separated ☐

PATIENT'S ADDRESS (No., Street) _109 West Central Ave._

City _Stephenson_   State _OH_   ZIP Code _60089_

HOME TELEPHONE (_614_) _022-3111_   SOCIAL SECURITY NUMBER _920_ _39_ _4567_

PATIENT'S RELATIONSHIP TO INSURED   Self ☒   Spouse ☐   Child ☐   Other ☐

ALLERGIES _____   REASON FOR VISIT _routine physical_

REFERRED BY _Dr. Janet Wood_

STUDENT STATUS   Full time ☐   Part time ☐   Non-student ☒

PATIENT'S OCCUPATION _manager_	SPOUSE'S OR PARENT'S NAME _____
EMPLOYMENT STATUS _full-time_	OCCUPATION _____
EMPLOYER'S NAME _Nichols Hardware_	EMPLOYER'S NAME _____
BUSINESS ADDRESS _____	BUSINESS ADDRESS _____
City _____ State _____	City _____ State _____
ZIP Code _____	ZIP Code _____
BUSINESS TELEPHONE _(614) 789-0200_	BUSINESS TELEPHONE _____
(Include Area Code)	(Include Area Code)

<table>
<tr><td colspan="3" align="center">PRIMARY INSURANCE PLAN</td><td colspan="2">IS THERE A SECONDARY HEALTH BENEFIT PLAN?</td></tr>
<tr><td colspan="2">PLAN NAME
Physicians' Choice Svcs.</td><td>PATIENT'S ID #
142395</td><td colspan="2" align="center">☒ YES   ☐ NO   *If yes, complete below.*</td></tr>
<tr><td colspan="3">POLICYHOLDER'S NAME (Last Name, First Name, Middle Initial)
Robertson, Stewart</td><td colspan="2">OTHER POLICYHOLDER'S NAME (Last Name, First Name, Middle Initial)
Robertson, Stewart</td></tr>
<tr><td colspan="3">POLICYHOLDER'S ADDRESS (No. Street)
same as above</td><td colspan="2">EMPLOYER'S NAME OR SCHOOL NAME
Nichols Hardware</td></tr>
<tr><td>CITY</td><td>STATE</td><td>ZIP CODE</td><td colspan="2">INSURANCE PLAN NAME OR PROGRAM NAME
USAHealth Hospitalization</td></tr>
<tr><td>% OF COVERAGE
80</td><td colspan="2">TELEPHONE (INCLUDE AREA CODE)
(   )</td><td colspan="2">SECOND POLICY'S GROUP NUMBER AND I.D. NUMBER
103955   920394567</td></tr>
<tr><td colspan="3">POLICYHOLDER'S GROUP AND SOCIAL SECURITY NUMBER
339U   920-39-4567</td><td colspan="2" rowspan="2">POLICYHOLDER'S DATE OF BIRTH   SEX
12 | 21 | 63   M ☒   F ☐
M   D   Y</td></tr>
<tr><td colspan="3">POLICYHOLDER'S DATE OF BIRTH   SEX
12 | 21 | 63   M ☒   F ☐
M   D   Y</td></tr>
</table>

Regardless of any insurance coverage I/we may or may not have, it is my/our responsibility to pay the entire bill. In the event that this office needs to obtain legal assistance in collection of any unpaid balance, I/we agree to pay costs and attorney fees, as allowable by law, and acknowledge receipt of a photocopy of this agreement.

I/we authorize the release of the above patient's medical records for billing purposes.

Stewart Robertson _____   _11/17/03_
Signature   Signature   Date

I/we authorize payment of medical benefits to the physician listed below.

Stewart Robertson _____   _Dr. Robert Beach_   _11/17/03_
Signature   Signature   Physician   Date

Index